Counseling the Communicatively Disabled and Their Families

(A Manual for Clinicians)

Second Edition

Counseling the Communicatively Disabled and Their Families

(A Manual for Clinicians)

Second Edition

George H. Shames, PhD

LEA LAWRENCE ERLBAUM ASSOCIATES, PUBLISHERS
2006 Mahwah, New Jersey London

Lawrence Erlbaum Associates, Inc., Publishers
10 Industrial Avenue
Mahwah, New Jersey 07430
www.erlbaum.com

Cover design by Kathryn Houghtaling Lacey

First edition published by Pearson Education, Inc.

Library of Congress Cataloging-in-Publication Data

Shames, George H., 1926–
Counseling the communicatively disabled and their families : a manual for clinicians / by George H. Shames. — 2nd ed.
p. cm.
Includes bibliographical references and index.
ISBN 0-8058-5743-5 (c. : alk. paper)
ISBN 0-8058-5744-3 (pbk. : alk. paper)
I. Title.

RC428.8.S53 2006
616.85′50651—dc22

2005049474
CIP

Books published by Lawrence Erlbaum Associates are printed on acid-free paper, and their bindings are chosen for strength and durability.

Printed in the United States of America
10 9 8 7 6 5 4 3 2 1

This book is dedicated
to my wife, Joan,
my partner in self-discovery
as a part of everyday living.

CONTENTS

ABOUT THE AUTHOR

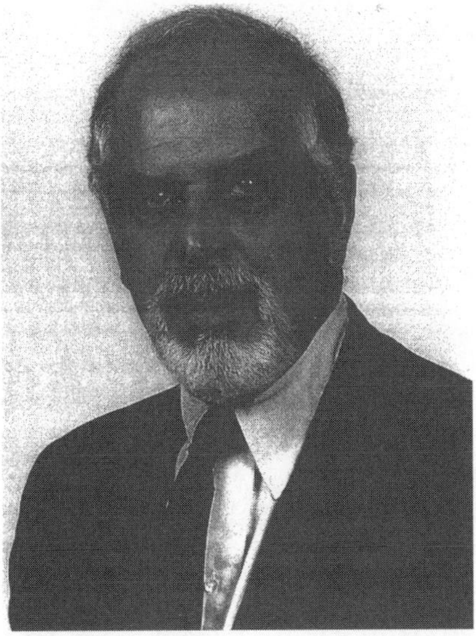

George H. Shames, PhD, is Professor Emeritus from the University of Pittsburgh. He is a licensed psychologist and a licensed speech pathologist. He has authored 11 books and has given lectures and workshops throughout the United States, Canada, Australia, Israel, Mexico, and Japan on the topics of stuttering and counseling.

PREFACE TO THE SECOND EDITION

One of the many benefits associated with publishing a second edition of a book is the opportunity it provides for revising. I wish to express my gratitude to the editors and to the current publisher for obtaining reviews of the first edition published by Allyn & Bacon that provided some very valuable guidance regarding appropriate changes that would constitute improvements in this, the Second Edition. Specific thanks are extended to Cathleen Petree, the sponsoring editor for Lawrence Erlbaum Associates, and to reviewers such as Jacqueline Hinckley, University of South Florida.

In this Second Edition, the reader is provided an expanded and detailed history of the pertinent literature, history, theory, and research that served as the basis for the format of the counseling procedures presented. The background, supportive literature was both updated and directly related to the actual counseling activities, beliefs, and attitudes to be learned.

This book integrates and brings together the theory, tactics, and history of operant conditioning and the principles of reinforcement of B. F. Skinner, and the theory, principles, and tactics of Client-Centered Therapy, regarding Self-Discovery and Self-Actualization developed by Carl Rogers. It also describes the evolution of Rogerian thought that extends beyond the realms of counseling and clients, and projects into everyday styles of human communication, in their natural contexts and circumstances.

In addition, the book integrates the principles and the theory of Authier and Ivy regarding Intentionality and client focus, as well as the processes of dimensionalizing specific counseling behaviors, which has come to be known as microcounseling. The ideas of Strupp regarding trust and affection are added to the process as yet another dimension of counseling that needs to be learned. These are the ideas that underlie the processes of counseling that are considered in this book.

The content is further expanded by calling your attention to the need to attend to multicultural issues that can be factors in the counseling process. The trust, the intimacy, the revelations, and the relationships that develop during counseling can easily be affected by specific family and ethnic beliefs, superstitions, and comfort levels, as well as by acceptance and understandings associated with different cultural backgrounds and experiences. Such variables need our attention, and, sometimes, further, in-depth anthropological education.

Finally, I wish to emphasize that counseling can only be learned by doing it. *Learning by doing* is a feature that is emphasized in this book via the many Suggested Practice Projects that are presented to enhance your acquisition of these skills.

All of this information and follow-up activity constitutes a major commitment on your part that in the long run will prove to be quite meaningful and valuable in both your professional and personal future.

PREFACE TO THE FIRST EDITION

When the poetry of the mind
Turns inward to embrace itself,
When its metered rhythms
Become echoes of its former grace,
When one alone means all alone
And the joys of living seem lost,
That is the moment
When the human spirit lingers
And reaches out to survive.
—ghS

Try to imagine living in a foreign country where you cannot communicate because you do not know the language. The visual and auditory alphabets are foreign. The sounds of the language convey no meaning to you. You cannot read, write, understand, or talk to anyone. Your communication system, your basic vehicle for social interaction, for developing interpersonal relationships, perhaps even your economic and physical independence may be in jeopardy. You may be the target of social penalties and even prejudice. The things that most of us take for granted are not available and become sources of stress for you. No friends, and limits on education and occupational potential, are a part of your everyday living.

Given such a scenario, how would you feel? At the very least, you would feel frustrated and exhausted from not being able to communicate. Anger and depression, as well as low self-esteem and low self-expectations and anxiety, might become a deeply embedded part of your life.

You might feel quite alone and isolated from the rest of the world around you.

This is not a far-fetched situation. Immigrants, refugees, and native-born citizens who have grown up with, and even as adults live with a communication problem live under such conditions and face such hardships.

Communication, by its very nature, is a system for social interactions that carries with it all of the emotional components of life. Having a communication disability does not immunize a person from the problems of everyday living, but rather does just the opposite. It targets such a person and makes him or her even more vulnerable to emotional problems. Therefore, communication problems, by definition, must include these interactive and emotional components, and therefore demand clinical and therapeutic attention.

Yet, if we engage in a quick perusal of the various definitions of specific communication problems, we see that most of the commentary deals with sensorimotor, neurophysiological, and anatomical content. As a result, most of the therapeutic tactics and most of the teaching of communication problem specialists focus on how to teach new communication skills to their clients. Very little attention is given to the communication–social interaction–emotional connections. There is acknowledgment that these connections exist, but not very much attention is paid to how and what to do about them.

This book deals with these connections. It also deals with how to learn the skills that are necessary to help the communicatively disabled deal with these interactive and emotional issues.

The information in this book starts with the basic elements of counseling. Although the exemplars relate to communication problems, these elements of counseling are appropriate for counseling across the broad spectrum of situations where people need help with what they believe, how they feel, how they interact, and how they deal with emotional stress. They therefore may have application in a basic way, no matter what the content and context of the situations might be. Learning how to listen, how to help people express their feelings, how to share your own experience, and how to interpret the client to himself are applicable to the human condition and applicable to the many issues of the human condition that all types of clinicians and helpers face with their clients.

We are indeed fortunate to have available to us the sensitivity, the genius, and the creativity of the many scholars, theorists, and researchers who have devoted their energies to understanding the very complex processes, organization, and repair of the human condition. I am referring here to those systems that govern our thoughts, beliefs, and feelings, which in turn influence and drive what we do and how we act.

The commentaries from these scholars about the integration of the body and mind, and about the relationships between the intellect and feelings and emotions, are sometimes philosophical, sometimes scientific, sometimes spiritual, and sometimes poetic. They have identified a unique beauty about the existence and integration of its parts as well as its totality as an orderly system, while also revealing a respect for its complex viability and vulnerability. They have sensitized us to both the overt and the covert nature of things, to the obvious and concrete and to the hidden and symbolic. Finally, they have provided a path, and guidance along that path, to the avenues of repair that might be available when these systems of thought and feelings are in need of help. We are indebted to these people for the basic foundations they have provided for our thinking. They outnumber by far the many who are named and acknowledged in this volume.

The author wishes to express his gratitude to several individuals and agencies who offered their help during the development and writing of this book.

Appreciation goes to the following reviewers for their comments on the manuscript: Richard J. Morris, Florida State University; Tanya Sue Enloe,Valdosta State University; and Joshua M. Gold, University of South Carolina.

Special thanks are offered to Audrey Holland, Amy Ramage, and Pelagie Beeson for their advice and guidance regarding counseling aphasic patients; to Kagan, Winckel, and Shumway of the York Center for Aphasia Rehabiltation in Ontario, Canada for the use of their film titled *Supportive Conversation;* to Larry Boles and Mimi Lewis, for making available a series of actual counseling sessions conducted with aphasics; to the class in Interviewing and Counseling during the summer of 1998 at Northern Arizona University (Tracy Adams, Judy Amadee, Brigette Bath-Barney, Wendy K. Burnett, Kelly DeBruin, Carol Julien, Marie Max, Andrea McGehee, Wendy Payne, Janet Usselman, Laurie Watson, and Tristan Young), for their willingness to participate in the execution of the contents of this manual, and for their feedback and suggestions to improve it. Each of them individually contributed in a unique way to the final product. Finally, my appreciation goes out to Gail Kilburg and Margy Forbes, my teaching assistants, and the hundreds of graduate students who were required to enroll in the course in Interviewing and Counseling during their matriculation at the University of Pittsburgh, for their feedback as they experienced and put into practice the various counseling tactics, behaviors, and training exercises described in this book.

1

INTRODUCTION

The purpose of this book is to help Speech and Language pathologists and audiologists learn the basics of counseling as it relates to communication problems.

It can be used either as a textbook for a formal class in Interviewing and Counseling, or as a manual for self-learning.

The specific behaviors and tactics considered are also applicable across the broad spectrum of diverse problems where group and individual counseling are appropriate.

Rarely do we enter into anything at its very beginning or exit at its conclusion. In any endeavor we may undertake we quickly realize that many others have been there before us and many others will be there after us, addressing the same or similar issues. With each ensuing layer of attention there is a resulting direct influence on what follows, and thus a direct bearing on the content and nature of this book.

There is Rogers (1942, 1979) for his original thinking and development of Client-Centered Therapy, and his ideas concerning warmth, empathy, genuineness, self-discovery, and self actualization; Rotter (1966), for his concepts of internal and external locus of control, which underlie so much of the basic thinking and research on counseling; Carkhuff and Berenson (1976) for their delineation of the special roles of helper and helpee and for their behavioral orientations for dimensionalizing the process of interviewing; Strupp (1962, 1972) for his writings about trust and love and the significance of the initial impact of the therapist on the total outcome of therapy; Matarazzo, Phillips, Wiens, and Saslow (1965) for defining the parameters of the interview and for their research on the significance of silence and therapist talking time during the interview; Truax (1967, 1972) for his research on the measurement of empathy and on the patient–therapist interaction; Ivey (1983) for his concepts of intentionality and the need to develop a repertoire of counseling skills; and Ivey and Authier (1978) for their ideas about how one might dimensionalize and integrate learnable behaviors into an effective set of interviewing and counseling skills.

A special acknowledgement is due to Ivey and Authier (1978) for emphasizing that interviewing and counseling can only be learned by doing; and to Skinner (1953) for his principles of reinforcement, which we will readily see enhance our understanding of the dynamics of the strengthening and weakening of thoughts, beliefs, and behaviors. These processes appear to function for both the client and the counselor through their verbal and nonverbal feedback to each other during interviews.

These are only a few of the many people who deserve acknowledgment. I have tried to note these many influences as much as possible and as space permits. I can only ask forgiveness from those who have been omitted.

There are many more whose research and ideas have influenced the content of this book. For those readers and scholars who are interested in a larger sample of the history of thought, theory development, and research, on the subject of counseling, we refer you to *Microcounseling*, by Ivey and Authier, to *The Dynamics of Interviewing*, by Kahn and Cannell, and to *The Anatomy of Psychotherapy*, by Lennard and Bernstein. They provide a more pervasive consideration of these many contributors than we have space for in this manual.

We realize that we enter in midstream, and can only hope that what we do with this brief clinical application manual may make things better for those who follow. It is this desire to reach those of you who wish to learn how to counsel the communicatively handicapped that has influenced the content, the organizational design, and the suggested strategies contained in this book.

Some of this book deals with specific interviewing and counseling behaviors, including their form and rationale as well as optimal timing for use during an interview. Attention is also given to how to learn and practice these skills so that they become a part of one's counseling repertoire. Other parts of the book deal with developing certain holistic attitudes and behaviors that may characterize the entire interview, and learning how to communicate these holistic attitudes to the client. The learning of these skills and attitudes is enhanced if they are considered one at a time, sometimes quite separate and independent of one another, and then are gradually integrated into the clinical interview.

The attitudes, behaviors, and communication of the counselor are the three underlying themes that are the central core of this book. Each of these categories of counselor characteristics targets two basic concepts. One is "focus on the client," which is both attitudinal and behavioral, and which demands the subordination of one's self. The other concept is "intentionality," which implies maximizing the counselor's control over what he or she does during a counseling interview, and minimizing his or her accidental, random, and nondeliberate behaviors.

These concepts of "focus" and "intentionality" will come up repeatedly in the progression of material that is presented. As you will see, they are the key for the development of all of the other facilitative and helpful attributes being considered. Also, it should be pointed out that there is no gender differentiation intended regarding the subject of the content, for either client or counselor. The use of such words as "his" or "her" are means to refer to both males and females, unless there is a differentiating comment in the content.

2

GETTING COMFORTABLE WITH COUNSELING

A number of issues must be considered during our immersion into the actualities of interviewing and counseling with the communicatively handicapped and their families.

One of these issues deals with our own comfort level, as speech, language, and hearing clinicians, relative to taking on the functions of a counselor.

Many of us see ourselves as being limited to only our primary functions of helping the communicatively handicapped change the way they communicate. As communication specialists we have a natural tendency to focus on our functions as a source of information, as diagnostician, prognosticator, and teacher of new communication skills. However, such an exclusive focus may be too narrow because it does not take into account the emotional sequalae associated with communication problems. Flasher and Fogle (2004) in their book *Counseling Skills for Speech-Language Pathologists and Audiologists*, pointed out that clients with communication problems can show a wide range of emotional problems. They specifically mention depression, guilt, fear, resistance, anger, and crises.

Issues of self-esteem, denial of a problem, motivation to change, acceptance of change in one's self, changes in interpersonal relationships, as well as conflicts between old and new self-expectations resulting from therapeutic change, can all be factors in therapy. In addition, educational, occupational, social, and interpersonal relationship issues commonly warrant examination in the context of living with a communication problem, as well as in the context of having changed how one communicates, or being free of their communication problem. Each of these issues has a powerful emotional underpinning that drives them to function either constructively or destructively in a person's life.

Wolf and Wolf (1975) in their *Counseling Skills Evaluation Manual* raised questions that we must take into account if we are to be effective.

They asked, What do people seek from a helping relationship? Many seek relief from painful symptoms; others wish to learn more adaptive and successful ways of living. At deeper levels, individuals hope to find serenity, peace of mind, and freedom from disabling conflicts. Many hunger to find meaning and purpose in life. Still others wish to become more productive and accomplish more of their ambitions. Expanding one's awareness, being more spontaneous, and becoming free from inhibitions are other goals for clients. Learning to be the master of oneself, effective at living, making important decisions about relationships, and becoming capable of commitment, intimacy, and genuineness are crucial issues at the core of life itself. How can people develop the means necessary to reach such heights of personal accomplishment and self-actualization?

Carkhuff (1969b), in addressing this question, has suggested that two processes are necessary for one to become more self-actualizing: *self-exploration* and *action*.

In order for a person to improve he must explore his behavior, thoughts, and feelings, as well as how he deals with stress, relates to others, and handles frustrating situations and disappointments. He must learn how to love in the profound sense of the word and discover his purpose in life.

As an individual explores himself, he learns more about his own self-image, his habitual behavior, and the way he interacts with others. As a result, he develops increasing self-awareness. Not only does a person gain insights as a result of self-exploration, but he also discharges pent-up emotions. Feelings associated with traumatic, painful, and personally embarrassing or damaging experiences in the past are relived, and the emotional reservoirs of painful experiences are released, thus producing freedom from the constrictions and conflicts that may have plagued the person.

Families and individuals living with communication problems are certainly not immune to these emotional issues in their lives. On the contrary, they experience more than their fair share of them because of their communication problems.

However, knowing the "whys" of one's behavior and experiencing freedom from painful emotions does not necessarily lead to lasting improvement. Individuals must do more than explore themselves in order to achieve enduring growth. They must take action. For individuals having communication problems, they are faced not only with the problem of learning new communication skills, or adjusting to living with some unchangeable aspect of their communication behavior, but also with the need to experiment with new behaviors and new techniques of living. They must put into operation new methods of reacting to others and dealing with frustrations. They must learn new ways of thinking about themselves and others. They must learn more effective techniques for living successfully. They must learn constructive behaviors to replace the former self-defeating, destructive behaviors—*a process that requires risk taking*. (p. 7)

Theodore Reik (1949) in his book, *Listening with the Third Ear* described an event that is most appropriate to this discussion, because it involved being encouraged to take a risk and to try something he had never done before.

When he was still a student studying with Freud, and walking home in the city of Vienna, Reik ran into "the great man" and told him about a problem he was having in making some decisions about marriage and his profession, hoping that Freud would give him some advice.

Freud stated,

> I can only tell you of my personal experience. When making a decision of minor importance, I have always found it advantageous to consider all the pros and cons. In vital matters, however, (with Freud not knowing the content of Reik's stress) such as the choice of a mate or a profession, the decision should come from somewhere within ourselves. In the important decisions of our personal life, we should be governed, I think by the deep inner needs of our nature. (p. vii)

Without telling him what to do, but incidentally mentioning the very content areas that were bothering Reik, Freud had helped him make his own decisions that stuck with him the rest of his life.

Counseling around such issues as decision making is one of the most common problems encountered by people, and the timeliness of Freud's sharing behavior is a powerful example of several strategies that a counselor might employ to be helpful in such a circumstance.

By virtue of our training, education, and clinical presence as communication specialists, we are uniquely positioned to consider such emotional problems.

But we must also consider how our teaching functions may either relate to or be kept separate from counseling.

Luterman (1977) and Rollin (1987), although 10 years apart from each other, reinforced the continuing importance of separating guidance counseling from psychological counseling. Luterman, in his 1977 book, which focuses on the hearing impaired, distinguished guidance counseling as a process that provides information to the client and to his or her family. This is a very important function, especially when the client is a newborn or a toddler. The parents need information about parenting a hearing-impaired child, and also about the process of aural habilitation and developing methods for their child to acquire communication skills. Unfortunately, far too often, such guidance counseling involving giving advice and information can become the only form of counseling made available to them. There are numerous psychological issues related to being hearing impaired or having the parental responsibilities for being helpful to one's child with such a problem. A different category of counseling, which has come to be known as psychological counseling, may be needed in addition to guidance counseling. This is also true for an individual who develops a hearing problem later in life. Adjusting to living with a hearing problem after many years of hearing normally can be a major source of stress that generates a feeling of social isolation.

Luterman (2001) has strongly recognized this often unmet need and takes the counseling process further and deeper into considering the emotional dimensions of living with silence.

Such clients need more than information and advice, and the audiologist might well take on such additional counseling responsibilities, if he or she obtains the appropriate education and clinical training.

Rollin (1987) also differentiated guidance counseling from psychological counseling, similar to the thinking of Luterman.

Using a medical model, Rollin pointed out that guidance counseling is more directive and involves providing information to a client, whereas psychological counseling involves helping a normal person to make appropriate adjustments. This can be in the form of client-centered counseling in which the client is encouraged to engage in self-discovery, examining oneself, and then developing and engaging in strategies to resolve stressful issues. He also pointed out that psychological counseling could also be directive wherein the counselor directs the client into certain beliefs and actions.

Rollin (2000) further pointed out that each of these types of counseling is far different from psychotherapy where the client is diagnosed as showing very abnormal psychological reactions, beliefs, feelings, and acts. He stated that psychological counseling is for normal people to help them solve problems and make readjustments for everyday living. Such counseling can help make adjustments rather than personality changes.

On the other hand, psychotherapy is for sick people who need to make personality changes because of psychological abnormalities.

Hutchinson (1979) suggested that the many different methods of counseling can be classified into five main categories. These would include (a) behavioral counseling, (b) client-centered counseling, (c) role playing, (d) psychoanalysis, and (e) drug intervention.

It is important that we define what counseling is, especially as it might differ from psychoanalysis or other forms of psychotherapy. There are significant differences between psychotherapy and counseling and important overlaps as well.

The most significant differences are that psychotherapy attempts to restructure the personality, especially in terms of a particular theoretical orientation about the nature and dynamics of personality. Psychotherapy generally views the client as being ill, and as a result searches for the cause or the theoretical etiology of a person's problems. The person's overall history, family relationships, and the reliving of early childhood trauma are viewed as keys to resolution.

Many psychotherapies have been developed and are being practiced in our society, each with a different focus on such things as cognitive experiences, precognitive experiences, the unconscious, the collective unconscious, personality archetypes, complexes, unconscious defense mechanisms, and levels of repression. Theoretical concepts include the ego, super ego, and id, as well as phases of psychological development (i.e., oral, anal retentive), and sexual conflicts. Each of these is an integral element in the theory, thinking, and tactics associated with these psychotherapies. Some of these therapies employ dream interpretation and free association as parts of their repertoire. Each embraces a psychodynamic orientation that underlies its therapeutic tactics.

Often psychotherapy treats the presenting complaint as an overt symptom of a much broader and more pervasive underlying problem. Thus, in therapy, the symptom soon loses its importance and significance. The focus then shifts from the symptom to the nature of the underlying problem, as stated in the theoretical dynamics of the client's personality.

Counseling, by contrast, deals with the present, with here and now strategies for coping with life, decision making, and current problems (Haan, 1977), instead of a medical illness approach, and uses a learning model whereby the counselor helps clients to become aware of themselves, of what they believe and feel, and how these things affect what they do and how they interact with society. Counseling can be quite directive, even when it is "person centered" (or considered nondirective). It is often related to specific types of situations such as in grief counseling, sexual counseling, educational counseling, pastoral counseling, marriage counseling, family counseling, or occupational counseling. Some of these approaches offer guidance and advice on what and how to think, what to believe, and how to act.

The overlap between counseling and psychotherapy comes primarily from the tactics used during clinical interviews, and not from their underlying theoretical dynamics or goals. There is much that the two fields share in terms of how counselors and therapists interact with clients. Many of the tactics we consider that relate to attitudes as well as to interviewing behaviors are characteristic of both counseling and psychotherapy. Even though they may differ significantly in their theoretical underpinnings, or in the dynamic process and goals of their particular therapy, they share and use the same or similar tactics and behaviors in the service of their unique dynamic processes and goals.

A third issue deals with the attitudes, values, beliefs, and self-awareness of the counselor, and how the counselor influences his or her clients. Client and counselor both learn many things about themselves as well as about each other during these sessions.

Among these things that each of them may be learning about each other are the many multicultural factors and issues that we live with in our multicultural society. When they arise they should not be ignored as they could become a significant factor in the relationship and in the overall counseling process. In some instances, it might be helpful to match the client and the counselor from the standpoint of gender, race, ethnic background, and cultural values. It could also be just as important to make sure that the participants do not match each other.

With regard to communication problems, it is known that different groups in different parts of the world differ sharply in their information and beliefs regarding certain kinds of communication problems, which could become an issue that requires attention in therapy.

For example, in some cultures a cleft palate or cleft lip is believed to be a punishment of parents for past sins. In some cultural groups, certain childhood communication problems are viewed very positively as a sign that this is a god- given gift for a special child. In other cultures there is great pride in verbal skills that would lead them to deny the existence of a problem or reject certain types of therapy that would require its public recognition. Some cultures believe that children should be seen but not heard. Such a cultural attribute could slow down language and communication development, and become a problem if such an attribute collides with cultures that value the opposite of that attribute in their children.

Values, superstitions, and beliefs could become active factors in counseling if the client feels that he or she has to protect his secrets, or his beliefs from his family, or friends, or even from the therapist and counselor. It would be well for someone who is trying to help to have some knowledge or background that would enable him or her to recognize any of these issues if they arise. These things vary from one community to the next and it could prove helpful to encourage the client to share this kind of information with you, without being judged or in fear of having to let go of things that may be quite important to him and to his or her family. The sharing of such issues, no matter how foreign to the thinking of the counselor, requires trust, understanding, and genuine acceptance from the counselor. As a way of getting started into such information it is recommended that you examine some introductory literature (see Payne & Taylor, 2000, chap. 4, "Multicultural Influences on Human Communication" in *Human Communication Disorders—An Introduction* edited by Shames and Anderson, 6th edition). Following that, some firsthand experiences with various multicultural populations could be most beneficial and applicable to your work. It could become a positive cultural adventure for both participants, if the counselor maintains his self-subordination role and permits the client to take the lead. But we should remain alert that such sharing by the client may be enhanced if the counselor takes the first risky step in trust by sharing some of his own cultural attributes as a way of encouraging his client to open the door into his most private thoughts and values.

For the counselor, there must always be a self-awareness, to insure that he is not inserting his own needs into the counseling. For the client there is an opportunity to learn the style and tactics and honesty and persistence of the counselor. In a sense the counselor often becomes a role model for the client from which the client learns the process of self-discovery. By doing to himself and for himself what he observes the counselor doing during the interviews, he can get in touch with his own beliefs, motivations, and feelings that enable him to take on more responsibility for maintaining therapeutic change.

There is also a major issue of adapting traditional counseling tactics that depend primarily on talking between a client and a counselor to populations who do not talk or have very limited language skills. Such populations as the neurologically involved or the elderly may need significantly different approaches to counseling.

Then there is the major issue of how one acquires the attitudes, the values, the emotional sensitivity, the behavioral skills, and the self-evaluative honesty and awareness that are essential for effective counseling.

This is related to an immediate issue for the reader and student of counseling who wants to learn how to do it. It is the issue of maintaining a commitment to do what has to be done in order to learn how to become an effective counselor. Reading about counseling can certainly be helpful and is a necessary part of your learning. However, merely reading about interviewing and counseling doesn't accomplish the entire job. It will become quickly apparent that *if you want to learn to counsel, you have to do it*; and the more you do it the better you become, and the more effective your counseling tactics become. This is a manual that helps you to learn to do things, to acquire certain attitudes and behaviors, to practice these behaviors in small steps, and that leads you into effective interviewing and counseling,

Therefore, in addition to its content, this manual organizes a series of practice projects and exercises that are the basic elements of counseling. They are patterned after the Ivey and Authier concepts of microcounseling (1978).

If you commit yourself to this process it is thought that you not only will improve your counseling skills, but you may find that much of what you do professionally may also influence your personal interactions. Each of these issues is addressed as we consider the various elements of interviewing and counseling.

As you progress through the content of this manual you will find specific Suggested Practice Projects associated with the attributes and behaviors under consideration.

These practice projects represent a sequence of experiences designed to get you started in learning the basic tactics, skills, behaviors, and principles of interviewing and counseling. They are just the beginnings, and will require many supervised and collaborative experiences in the interviewing and counseling processes addressed. They represent the start of a long journey of learning, involving brief, mock interviews, as well as extended practice counseling sessions, and eventually very real counseling sessions that will continue long after you have completed the reading and practice exercises offered in this manual. During this journey you will gradually accumulate the experiences necessary for fine-tuning the skills acquired from these introductory lessons.

The first time you engage in these practice projects they should be addressed sequentially, and in connection with the particular content you are dealing with in this manual, in the order that it is presented. You should stay on the same practice project until you show growth and progress, before moving onto the next content area and its associated practice projects.

Such a commitment on your part requires that you arrange for several things to happen that will enable you to learn and progress through this book. These are (a) acquire a high quality audiotape recorder and several audiotapes, (b) special practice projects are suggested at appropriate times as they relate to the content under consideration. They will typically involve conducting short interviews to practice specific microcounseling behaviors that will be integrated into longer 1-hour interviews on a weekly basis. You will need to recruit two interviewing partners that you can practice with in different ways. One of these partners is for brief practice projects, the other is for engaging in real counseling sessions on a weekly basis. These interviews are to be audiotape recorded or videotaped for your later review and analysis.

Ideally the person who engages in these brief practice projects with you might be a classmate in your course. It should not be the person who has volunteered to be your long-term interviewing partner.

If you are using this manual in a formal class, you will be engaging in a number of practice exercises with classmates that enables you to learn and practice specific tactics, one at a time. There will be role playing and brief interviewing sessions that focus on a process known as successive approximations. This means that you will learn to do your counseling, one tactic at a time, and gradually build one tactic onto another one, until you are engaging in a larger, more pervasive, and "real" process of counseling with one of your classmates.

You will probably reverse roles, so that one of you may serve as the "counselor" and one as the "client" on different occasions.

Whichever way you arrange for the occasions for your practice sessions, whether involving a large group such as a class, with a classmate during the class, or alone with interviewing partners, it should be made explicitly clear that what is said and heard remains confidential. It stays where it took place, and the name of any outside interviewing partner is never revealed. It should be pointed out that the content is never to be talked about, except for occasions appropriate to classroom discussion, but never outside of that classroom situation. Even then, identities remain confidential. As these practice sessions develop, the participants will no doubt do a lot of spontaneous sharing and revealing of things that are of importance to them, some of which they might consider to be quite personal and intimate. They need the assurance that what they say goes no further, and will not come back to haunt them.

Our experiences with these types of practice exercises have been extremely positive. The participants, as they practice and exchange roles, have stated that they learn the counseling tactics more effectively when the partner in the role of the "client" is relating truth rather than fiction. When the feelings and circumstances that are discussed are based on actualities, rather than "made-up" material, they report that they can both really "get into" the process and "learn more and learn better."

One of the results of the mock interviews being reality based is that the participants experience "trust" and "focus" between them. "Trust" becomes a personal, first-hand concept, rather than an academic abstraction.

If you are using this manual in a self-learning fashion, you should recruit someone who can function as your partner for these brief, practice sessions. The same benefits accrue as for the classroom situation.

Lastly, (c) you also need to acquire a long-term interviewing partner, preferably someone you do not know very well and do not spend time with socially. Ideally, this person should be available to you to interview 10 to 12 times, on a schedule of at least once a week. The time, place, and purpose of these sessions are limited to the purpose of conducting a counseling interview. They are not for casual social interactions and chitchat. If possible the location should be relatively quiet and free from interruption. Also, if possible, it should be in a neutral location where either party can feel free to leave if that becomes warranted.

Recruitment of an interviewing partner should be done as soon as possible, and you should conduct your first 1-hour interview with that person before reading the next chapter. This will provide you with a pretraining sample of your interviewing skills and will be used as a baseline against which you can evaluate any changes or progress you make in acquiring interviewing skills. Put this first taped interview in storage, and evaluate it later, after you have become familiar with how to evaluate yourself.

In approaching someone to serve as your interviewing partner, you should emphasize that you need their help in order to learn how to interview and counsel. You might tell them that you are not viewing them as neurotic or in need of counseling, but point out that we all face "decision making" in our lives and sometimes people benefit from talking about decisions they are facing; and that in addition to the help he is providing you, he may also benefit from doing this with you.

It is desirable to do these 10 to 12 interviews with the same interviewing partner, but not with a classmate with whom you interact during the class. The idea behind doing this with someone that you do not spend much time with is to minimize the interviewee's self-editing and fear of breaches of confidentiality. Doing the interviews with the same person will enable you to evaluate any changes in your counseling tactics, as well as changes in your interviewing partner as a function of the relationship that may develop between the two of you over that period of time that he or she is seeing you. Your contact with your partner should be limited only to the counseling session during the time he or she is serving as your long-term interviewing partner.

On a number of occasions you may find yourself referring to material that was discussed at an earlier time, with both your short-term and long-term interviewing partners. Or you may find it valuable to study and analyze interviews with both types of partners. When these practice interviews go beyond being short, brief, dissected practice activities, but instead take on the character of an actual interview, it is a good idea to tape record them for your future reference.

These are the immediate commitments and arrangements that should be made in order to proceed through this manual and to acquire the counseling behaviors under consideration.

Examine Tables A.I, A.II, and A.III, which appear in Appendix A. These tables provide a format for tracking various attributes and behaviors associated with clinical interviewing. They can be used by yourself to make judgments about your interviewing and counseling, or by others who observe your interviewing. It is your score sheet for charting progress in learning interviewing behaviors, so that you can see where you were compared to where you are or might be going. It can be useful for identifying strengths and weaknesses and areas that need attention and discussion. Make copies of these forms, because you will need a separate form for each interview you conduct.

On the front of the form are spaces for tabulating the frequencies of various specific counseling behaviors that you executed during the interviews you conduct. There are also rating scales for judging the presence or absence of certain facilitative and nonfacilitative attributes that might characterize large segments of the interview, or of the entire interview. You should tabulate and rate yourself on these scales as soon after the interview as possible.

On the reverse side of the form you should write down your impressions of the interview, including the various themes that were discussed by your interviewing partner as well as anything unusual, or events that may have caught your attention during the interview, including your own emotional reactions to anything that may have been talked about. These qualitative impressions may be an important source of information for tracking any changes that may be occurring with your partner as well as with yourself in any cumulative way. Possible topics to observe are your own focus, the development of trust and affection, and the occurrence of any uncontrolled emotional outbursts.

3

THE RELATIONSHIP BETWEEN SPEECH/LANGUAGE/HEARING THERAPY AND COUNSELING

Cataloguing each of the significant elements in managing communication problems is partly what this book is about. These various elements may come from different perspectives and acquire their clinical significance from the context of their applications.

At one point we may concern ourselves with such specific processes as reinforcement for learning new communication skills, or for learning the dynamics of speaking or producing sounds. At another point we may concern ourselves with nonspecific counseling processes such as the client's motivation, or the clinician–client relationship. We cannot identify any type of hierarchy among these perspectives and elements, nor do we wish to say that one element is more important than another. Speech and language therapy on the one hand and counseling on the other hand may interact with and depend on one another, or combine and function in concert with one another. Or they may be different ways of looking at the same events.

In addition, what we refer to as "the counseling interview" provides a pertinent illustration of a very complicated integration of "specific clinical–behavioral elements of counseling," and of "nonspecific, clinical, holistic elements" of counseling.

We are going to dissect "the interview" to heighten our awareness of these elements, with the full recognition that such a dissection will distort the process as it is holistically used and perceived. But we will look at its parts, try to understand its elemental workings and then attempt to put it all together again, so that ultimately like the watchmaker with a watch or the auto mechanic with the car, the final result will be a more effective total unit, and a user will be more knowledgeable, and more sensitive to self-correction.

The interview is the vehicle for developing the clinical relationship and its associated interactions. What is an interview? Matarazzo (1971) stated that "the interview is a form of conversation wherein two people, and recently more than two, engage in verbal and nonverbal interaction for the purpose of accomplishing a previously defined goal . . ." (p. 895). The issues, the skills, and the attitudes we will be considering are just as applicable to groups as they are to one-on-one situations.

Most of us think we know how to interview people, and most of us engage in it with little or no formal training. This is probably because there is so much overlap between the things we do during normal, everyday personal conversations and the things we do during an interview.

Also it may be due to the fact that there is no one right way to interview someone. However, unlike our typical interpersonal conversations that we have with friends, an interview has some very special properties that make it a special type of conversation.

Matarazzo (1971) pointed out that the interview has a fairly well-defined set of purposes for the interviewer and for the interviewee. These purposes may not necessarily coincide, nor remain the same for the participants. Purposes can range through such things as evaluating or diagnosing, defining a problem area more sharply, planning treatment strategies, establishing a working relationship, being emotionally supportive, giving information, or solving a problem.

The interview involves a "focus" on just one of the participants: the interviewee. The needs, the issues, and the problems of the interviewee dominate. The agenda of content, of what may be important to examine and explore at the moment, requires a focus on the other person. It is not a mutual exchange or sharing or expression of each other's needs. The needs of the interviewer are not the issues of primary concern here, unless they interfere with focusing on the interviewee. The role of the interviewer is to facilitate the interviewee's self-exploration, verbal expression, and an examination of thoughts and feelings about important and personal matters that may be causing problems for the interviewee. This process of focusing on the other person, and subordinating oneself, and the process of looking at oneself (the interviewer) as someone who may facilitate or impede the thoughts, feelings, and actions of another person, is very unlike our everyday conversations and interactions, and make the interview a unique and special arrangement between people. In this sense, it is a very one-sided, nonmutual relationship. One person expresses, reveals, and examines while the other facilitates the process.

When we look at how we function as communication specialists, we immediately see that interviewing is one of the basic vehicles for all of our endeavors. We talk to our clients and they talk to us. This goes on with children, adults, parents, and spouses, individually and in groups. It goes on whether we are helping to change articulation, eliminate a hoarse voice, establish speech that is free of stuttering, or helping a child to acquire and use language. Each of these particular speech therapeutics may emphasize different aspects of interviewing from problem to problem, from person to person, or at different times with the same person. But there is one attribute of the interview that is common to all. Purposes may vary, specific tactics may vary, but client focus does not.

To underscore some other of these common attributes further we should look at the larger perspectives of what we hope to accomplish in therapy for communication problems.

We are sought out to be of help to people who may or may not have a communication problem. We are sought out by people who think that they or members of their family should change the way they are. Sometimes these changes are major incursions in a behavioral sense. But often, even minor changes in speaking behavior may involve major emotional overtones. Changing the way we are is of necessity a profound, awesome, and often difficult and painful experience. It is tampering with our basic self-identity. Letting go of who we are or the way we were can be fraught with both fears and pain: pain over the past and fears about the future. It almost seems as though we go through a grieving or mourning for that part of ourselves that we are putting aside before we can comfortably embrace a new identity for our future. Perhaps the most dramatic illustration of this is the physical, emotional, and attitudinal changes that transsexuals experience as they anticipate and overtly become members of the opposite sex. But the behavioral, emotional, and self-identity changes of stutterers who become fluent, of falsetto males who become baritones, and of children who correct their articulation are in their own ways just as profound to these individuals. When we as clinicians accept the responsibility for helping someone to change the way he or she is, we are accepting more than the responsibility to help bring about a change in talking behavior. We are also accepting the responsibility for helping the person with the impact of that behavioral change and its integration within his total self-identity. People are more than the way they talk, and permanently changing the way they talk involves more than the things they do with their vocal mechanisms.

Communication problems develop and exist in the context and milieu of living, breathing, thinking, believing, and feeling human beings. They exist in the context of human social interactions, in the private feelings of the families and individuals who live with these problems day in and day out all of their lives. It is obvious that communication problems are multidimensional.

Reiterating the nature of this multidimensionality in our clients may make us more comfortable with seeing ourselves as being multidimensional helpers as well.

A communication problem is more than the way a person talks. We are here reducing such problems into dimensions that provide us with ways for approaching our tasks of helping people change the way they communicate. There are anatomical and neurophysiological dimensions, and sensorimotor dimensions. There are cortical dimensions of intelligence, linguistics, and memory. There are social interaction and cultural dimensions that may well define what is normal or acceptable, and there are emotional dimensions that the speaker and his family, and his listeners bring to the process of living with this type of problem. It is all part of being human. Although these many dimensions interact with each other, and although we sometimes dissect ourselves in order to understand ourselves, individuals respond and interact, not as separate, compartmentalized dimensions of themselves, but as a totality. Their communication problem is integrated into how they see themselves, how they define themselves, how they feel and think and interact as a total human being. It is therefore incumbent that we as clinicians respond with more than our teaching function, with more than our reinforcing functions, or our diagnostic and prognostic functions as speech and hearing and language experts. But given our unique training and experience with communication problems, we are in the best position to try to deal with as much of the totality as we can. This is not to deny the importance of surgeons, neurologists, psychiatrists and psychologists and educational planners in their roles as helpers, but it does strongly suggest that we can have a larger role than helping someone change the dynamics of their communication behavior. This becomes especially relevant when we deal with transferring communication skills learned in the therapy room to the client's real world of social and communication interactions.

Counseling focuses on the emotional and feeling components of communication problems, and deals with the emotional impact of therapy and the consequences of changing the way they are, of changing how they talk, and of changing how they interact with people. In some instances we may have to help someone learn to accept and live with the status quo, as in permanent physical damage or impaired brain functioning, which can occur in brain trauma, strokes, and paralysis.

Some of us would lump all of our functions, both as a person who helps someone change the way they communicate as well as someone who helps a client feel better about himself, under the term "counseling."

Giving advice and guidance about how to wear and use a hearing aid is directive teaching, and has come to be known as counseling. Telling the parents of a retarded child what they dread to hear about their child in terms of the future and advising them as to what they should do, is very directive information giving. It also has come to be known as counseling. Are these "directive" counseling functions of informing, teaching, and advising different from the more "client-centered" counseling that focuses on processes of self-discovery and self-actualization; on issues of self-esteem, valuing oneself, helplessness, fear, despair and feeling sorry for oneself, to name just a few of the issues that sometimes accompany a communication problem? The answer is a very loud "*YES.*" This is not merely a semantic or labeling issue. A very real question is whether a clinician can be the directive authority figure one moment, and then shift to become a listener who encourages self-discovery by the client by sharing his innermost feelings to you in the next moment. This is a shift for both the clinician and the client. Both must become aware of and become comfortable with this dramatic shift, back and forth, again and again, during interviews, for each of them.

It can be difficult for both the client and the clinician. And yet this is what is required, and this is part of the process. An awareness of what we are doing with regard to who takes the lead, the client or the clinician, concerning different issues in therapy, may have a direct bearing on how responsible the client eventually becomes for managing his new communication skills, as well as managing his other life changes after his therapy has terminated.

Both types of activities (directive and client centered) are valuable and necessary for an optimum regime of therapy, and their timing during therapy could be an important factor. You do not give up your overall functioning as a communication specialist when you engage in counseling, but you might delay some aspects of it or defer to a moment of counseling if only because of the sensitive nature and unpredictability of the moment when emotional issues might be presented to you by the client. For example, if your client has learned some new communication skill or behavior, and makes a speech error while talking to you about his fears of seeking a new job, it might be well to forgo correcting his speech or calling attention to speech errors at that moment, and instead concentrate on the content of what he is talking about. The timing of each kind of concentration, and the alternating of roles can become tricky, but with experience you soon learn to recognize what is appropriate for a particular and specific instant in time and context.

4

THE CLINICAL RELATIONSHIP

In *Reverence for Life* (1965), Albert Schweitzer said: "A man must not try to force his way into the personality of another. To analyze others—unless it be to help back to a sound mind someone who is in spiritual or intellectual confusion—is a rude commencement, for there is a modesty of the soul which we must recognize, just as we do that of the body" (pp. 6–7).

The principles, processes, and ethics of counseling must especially take into account Schweitzer's words of warning because counseling is such an intrusion into a person's modesty. But it is an intrusion whose mission is to restore, and while doing so, to preserve the dignity, self-respect, and well-being of the person in need.

Sometimes all we do is listen, and permit the informants to tell their story about their problems as they see them. Often that may be the most important thing we do. Sometimes we interpret and restate what they tell us by providing them with new information about their problems. Sometimes we help clients learn new skills, new ways of thinking and believing things about themselves. Sometimes we help them change the way they talk and communicate and interact with society. These are all necessary and legitimate functions. But underlying these several functions is a very basic and important thing that we must remember; we are in a special relationship with our clients. We are there to help; we have no other purpose. If this special relationship is to be effective, we need to do those things that will encourage the client to trust us. It is because of their trust that the clients open themselves up to us, permit us to teach them, and let us see into their most private fears, motivations, and anxieties that often accompany having a communication problem. Often these emotional components of a communication problem seriously affect the rate of therapeutic change, the duration of such changes, and how well the clients and their families can cope with these changes. It is only with their trust that we can be of maximum help.

Strupp (1972) suggested several factors that operate to make a patient susceptible to the influences of a therapist and therefore able to change. He mentions motivation, the distress of the patient, and early childhood experiences, in the forms of defense mechanisms against powerful, loving, judgmental, and trusted parents. He characterized psychotherapy (and it is equally applicable to counseling people with communication problems) in part as a patient's struggle against trusting the therapist; and in return the therapist's activities are designed to undermine these defenses against trusting him. Strupp further pointed out that trusting the therapist is a form of submission, a blind faith in the trustworthiness or basic goodness of the other person, and an abiding conviction that the other person will not use the power that the patient has been forced to place in his hands against the patient, except for "therapeutic purposes." Such submission can be painful because it can be risky for the client. We might even think of the therapist as engaging in the "art of gentle pain" in this process of submission, and, as Strupp stated, think of therapy as a series of lessons in basic trust. Strupp felt that in the final analysis the patient changes out of love for the therapist.

When we accept a client for speech therapy, to help bring about desirable changes in communication behavior, we are also accepting the responsibility for generating that person's trust to facilitate these changes. Generating and accepting a person's love and trust is not a casual or unimportant aspect of our work. Rogers (1972) has pointed out that the most difficult emotional expressions to facilitate in clients are the positive ones of love, affection, and trust. It would seem to follow then that their rejection and abuse is the most devastating to the human spirit.

In the clinical context, the violation of a client's trust could be a mortal blow to the clinical relationship and therefore to the entire process of therapy. This special kind of relationship is somehow accomplished through the tactics and processes of the interview. It is through a number of specific and nonspecific interviewing tactics, behaviors, and attitudes that the clinician can communicate his genuine concern for the well-being of the client individually, or for a group of clients if it is a group situation. It is also through the interview that both the client and the clinician eventually learn to let go of each other, even in this special relationship, as the client grows and becomes independent of his special therapeutic needs. The client, during his interviews, also learns to put therapy aside, as a part of the way he was. It may well be that unless these processes occur during clinical interviews, any of our other behavioral tactics in therapy, involving conditioning and reinforcement, may have only limited effects in the transfer and maintenance of new communication skills.

From time to time, as you read this book, you will be asked to place yourself in the shoes of your client, to become aware not only of yourself, but aware of your clients and the nature of their experiences with you. You have to learn to do this without injecting your own needs into this special situation.

Think for an instant, and react to this question: "How many people in this world do you trust? I mean trust in a total sense, with no inhibitions about what you might share with them, without fear of being judged or penalized for what you say or feel or believe?"

Some people feel that they can trust only superficial information about themselves to most of the people they know. There may be a special category of very few people to whom you might trust certain categories of information and feelings, like discussing your occupational goals with your parents, or your attitudes toward people you like or dislike, with a friend. Then there may be more intimate kinds of things regarding love and sex and hate and fears and guilt and embarrassment, that may involve one special friend. And then there may be certain honesties about yourself, your very human qualities, sometimes the things you are ashamed to admit that you have thought, or felt, or done, that you choose to admit to no one. These are the things that are reserved only for yourself.

What would have to happen that would enable you to entrust everything to someone? If you think about this for a moment, of all the people you know, are there any that you could trust in this way? Yet this is what we are asking of a client! You can't just say to your client "Don't worry, you can trust me with anything."

I want to suggest a few things that are essential for that kind of trust to take place.

1. You must be seen as someone who values and cares about the person.
2. You must be seen as being nonjudgmental, and not pronouncing what is right and what is wrong about what the client tells you.
3. You must be viewed as able to maintain confidentiality, so that the content of those things being shared does not come back to haunt or embarrass the client.

How do we go about gaining the trust of the client that will result in an effective therapeutic working relationship?

Probably the most important issue is being able to let the client know that he or she is important to you, in fact that he or she is the most important person in the world during those moments that you spend together.

Second, it is important that you understand how they feel and that you communicate your understanding to your client. Third, you should not be judgmental about anything clients tell you about themselves.

What you have to work with in yourself is your basic attitude toward your client, your listening skills, your eye contact, your body language and nonverbal behavior, and what you say.

All aspects of this relationship are unique and special: the people, the reasons for meeting, the time, the place, the duration and the roles that each one plays in it. This relationship does not have a socially mutual function, as with a friend or relative. It exists for the person in need of your help, and for no other reason; and these parameters should be established and clearly understood by all parties involved.

The way to open the door to being viewed as the kind of person who can be trusted is through your close, active listening. This is a learnable behavior that we discuss in greater detail later.

In order to accomplish these different and necessary multidimensional functions we learn to walk a very narrow, tight line. On the one hand we are viewed as being a very directive authority figure who is an expert about communication problems, and on the other hand we are seen as a nonauthoritative, person-centered counselor who helps the client engage in self-discovery relative to the emotional and socially interactive impacts of these communication problems. Our goal is to help him assume more and more responsibility for his own well-being and processes of change relative to how he communicates, as well as how he feels and interacts with society.

Accepting the fact that a person needs to change something about himself is a significant and often stressful experience. It precedes the actual process of changing the way he is, changing how he does things, and changing how he sees himself. Each of these stages of change is fraught with stress. It is no small task, and it carries with it the feelings and emotions of everyone who might be affected by these changes.

Again, let's take a moment for empathizing. Did you ever decide that there is something that you wanted to change about yourself? Did you talk about it, keep it a secret, do it alone, become part of a group? This decision to change is a major step. Doing something about it is even more difficult. Have you tried to lose weight, considered cosmetic surgery, considered using a hairpiece, or dealt with various addictions like smoking, sex, or substance abuses, considered divorce, occupational changes, even selling a house, or moving to another part of the country? If any of these changes are familiar to you then you already know how hard a process this can be. The same is true for the person having a communication problem that carries so many social and emotional penalties. The sense of helplessness and devaluing one's self can be overwhelming.

You have to be a very special person for the client to let you all the way in. Both of you are special in this regard. But it is not just the people in this context who are special, it is the context itself. It is a relationship that is unlike any other relationship either of you will participate in. It is not like a friendship. It is not mutual. Each of you has a role. The focus is on the client, and on helping the client. The client has to see this, and be helped to accept this. The counselor, even with his own self-awareness, has to subordinate himself and his own needs to that focus of being a helper. Both the counselor and the client have to recognize these differing roles of each, and realize when the clinician is functioning as a teacher, and when he is functioning as a counselor, when the session changes back and forth from being a student–teacher relationship to being a person-centered counselor–client relationship.

5

THE COUNSELING INTERVIEW

The counseling interview is the basic vehicle for learning to counsel. Talking about counseling in the abstract can be valuable, just as reading about counseling can be valuable. But actually engaging in counseling, and engaging in self-analysis, as well as analyses by colleagues, makes the process a reality, and gets you in touch with the actualities of what you are doing.

It is during the interview that the client experiences the human qualities of the clinician as well as her behavioral technological competence. As Fromm-Reichman stated about psychotherapy, the patient "needs an experience not an explanation" (in Strupp, 1962, p. 582).

Although learning to counsel comes from doing it, an understanding of what went into the development of what you are learning to do is extremely important, because it enables you to cope with the complexities that can emerge during the learning and engaging in these skills.

In one of the most memorable debates in the history of psychology, Carl Rogers and B. F. Skinner discussed a number of controversial issues concerning the control of human behavior (Rogers & Skinner, 1956, in *Science*, Vol. 124, pp. 1056-1066). They agreed that man generally has tried to predict and control human behavior. They also agreed that a science of human behavior is essential to understanding that behavior. The major differences between them involved who is doing the controlling, and who is being controlled. They strongly disagreed about how free a person generally is to make choices.

Skinner suggested that man is always under the control of external forces from the culture, from family, and from many externally imposed belief systems. These external forces provide the consequences for man's behavior, which either reinforce or weaken it.

On the other hand, Rogers recognized that man is only partially controlled by external forces, by what he termed "an external locus of control" (Rotter, 1966). This external locus of control is operating in psychotherapy, in the forms of reinforcement and punishment, which are under the control of the psychotherapist. By saying "yes" and "uhhuh" the therapist focuses the client on certain content and increases the frequency with which the client talks about that content. By saying "no" or "I don't understand" or not saying anything at all, the therapist may verbally and nonverbally punish certain content, and as a consequence the client reduces the frequency of that content. However, the major disagreement seems to be related to Rogers' explanation that the therapist is exercising his external control with the goal of having the client take over control of himself, and that the client develops a subjectively controlled "internal locus of control." The development of this subjective "internal locus of control" is an integral and pivotal part of client-centered therapy. The processes of self-discovery and self-actualization require that the therapist withdraws his control over the client as the client learns to exercise control over himself.

Skinner did not accept this concept of self-discovery and self-actualization as a subjective experience. He believed that the operation of external controls from society take the place of the controls that are eventually withdrawn by the therapist.

Skinner and Rogers also disagreed on issues surrounding the goals of controlling behavior, with Skinner stating that the goals are independent of the scientific process of control, whereas Rogers stated that the process is vulnerable to misuse and therefore the goals have to be explicitly related to the processes of control.

Both points of view, the one by Skinner and the one by Rogers, have interesting evolutionary histories.

On the one hand Skinner started his work in the laboratory conducting highly controlled experiments primarily with animals to test certain hypotheses regarding his theories of reinforcement and operant conditioning. In its most simple formulation he theorized that people learned to do certain things as a function of the consequences that their behavior generated. Positive reinforcement (a positive consequence) resulted in an increase in the frequency of the behavior that it followed.

Negative reinforcement was also a process of increasing the frequency of behavior because the consequence resulted in the termination of some ongoing aversive stimulation. Skinner also studied the effects of punishment and extinction as ways of reducing behavior. These laboratory studies were also carried out on human beings. They proved to be so promising that the concepts and tactics of reinforcement and conditioning were gradually taken out of the highly controlled laboratory situation and applied to a number of different types of human problems in institutions and in clinical settings, in controlled research studies throughout the United States.

Skinner himself offered an explanation as to how human language developed in terms of his ideas regarding operant conditioning in a book titled *Verbal Behavior* (1957).

Diagnostic audiology employed positive reinforcement as part of their audiometric examinations, and social environments were arranged in communities and hospitals for the mentally retarded, involving reinforcement contingencies for appropriate social interactions.

Krasner (1961, 1963) summarized much of the thinking and research regarding reinforcement of verbal behavior in psychotherapy.

Salzinger and Pisoni (1957) demonstrated that the frequency of affective verbal responses by schizophrenics during clinical interviews could be increased through verbal reinforcement tactics by a psychotherapist.

Greenspoon (1955) demonstrated the reinforcement of two spoken words simply by the consequence of two spoken sounds.

In a series of studies with people who stutter, Shames (1969) and Shames and Egolf (1976) demonstrated the application of principles of operant conditioning within the context of clinical interviews. They demonstrated that it was possible to strengthen (increase the occurrence of) desirable content as a consequence of verbal approval and weaken (decrease the occurrence of) undesirable content of what stutterers talked about during clinical interviews, as a consequence of verbal disapproval—with associated changes in overt stuttering behavior.

In another study Shames and Honeygosky (1976) showed that the number of affective, emotionally loaded statements made by a stutterer could be increased by positive reinforcement in the form of verbal approval provided by an interviewer following each such statement during clinical interviews. In yet another study, Shames and Johnson (1976) demonstrated that the frequency of comments by stutterers that indicated "decisiveness and goal setting" could be increased when it generated preplanned verbal approval from a clinician during a series of interviews.

During a slightly earlier time, but eventually overlapping the Skinnerian evolutionary history, a parallel evolutionary history was created by Carl Rogers in the area of counseling. In 1942, Rogers publicly introduced his ideas regarding nondirective therapy in his book titled *Counseling and Psychotherapy*. At the time of the beginnings of these parallel histories it seems improbable that either Skinner or Rogers could have anticipated that their ideas, theories, and tactics might collide and possibly become integrated with each other.

A chapter from Roger's 1942 book was republished in another book titled *Stuttering Then and Now* by Shames and Rubin (1986), with a significant updating postscript added by Julius Seeman, a cohort of Rogers. Some 44 years after Rogers introduced his ideas about nondirective therapy, Seeman described how the concepts of Rogers had undergone significant changes. Seeman characterized Rogerian thought as going through a three-stage evolutionary history.

It started with the ideas of nondirective therapy, moved on to a second stage known as client-centered therapy, and is now into its current stage of person-centered approach.

Seeman stated that the name of the first stage, nondirective therapy, made sense because it was seen as an antithesis to "directive therapy."

The early development on Roger's part was very much an empirical rather than a theory-based process. On the basis of his clinical experience, he had come to see that clients had surprising possibilities for exploring and comprehending their own areas of pain, but there was no body of knowledge and certainly no research that supported such a premise. These elements were to come later. It placed a strong emphasis on verbal technology.

Seeman pointed out that as new levels of understanding emerged, the earlier contrast themes against directive therapy were no longer necessary, and the term "nondirective" was less functional. The term "client centered" emerged, which described in more precise and affirmative terms the essence of this therapy. Seeman stated that its new title, "client centered" described with simple accuracy exactly what the core of the therapy was meant to be; namely, an approach in which the therapist centered attention on the world of the client's immediate experiencing. It focused on the internal frame of reference of the client. Along with this second stage of Rogerian thinking was a parallel theory of personality development, and a relationship between theory and therapy.

There are several dimensions to this theory and its relationship to the therapy. One deals with the relative emphasis on preconceptual experiencing on the one hand and cognitive processes on the other. The second dimension deals with the extent to which the therapist introduces structure into the therapeutic task. The phenomenon of "experiencing" is essential to personality change. Client-centered therapy has evolved a technology designed to facilitate the experiencing process in the client.

In its third stage of evolution, the client-centered approach recognized that the therapeutic approach described by Rogers need not be limited to therapy, but in fact had generic qualities. The elements of the therapeutic applications were seen to be constructive and enhancing, not only in therapy but in many other kinds of interpersonal settings. Although this recognition was voiced as early as 1951 in the development of the client-centered therapy by Rogers, it became strongly expanded by Rogers in the 1960s when Rogers left academia and moved into a community setting, the Western Behavioral Sciences Institute. In this setting, there were no clients, or people in need of help, but rather opportunities to apply these principles that were originally developed for applications to therapy could also be applied to interpersonal interactions and encounters. The term client-centered was no longer appropriate, and it gave way to the term "people centered." It has since been applied to issues with parents, in industry, in government, to theories and tactics of education, and even to conflict resolution in international relations. It has even reached the point where in some instances, Skinnerians and Rogerians have embraced the ideas of each other in dealing with and understanding the many challenges that have been presented to them in their various human adventures. In some instances researchers and clinicians have added their own creative thinking to the basic ideas of these two men.

Some of these activities have been in the form of clinical applications and research projects that have had powerful impacts on future research and broad and diverse real-life applications. The references contained in this book for the most part are the consequences of the thinking of these two men. And in turn, these spin-off projects with Skinner and Rogers at their core constitute the very basic foundation for the content of this book.

For purposes of analysis and evaluation as well as for learning, we can compartmentalize the attributes of the counseling interview into two general categories. One category can be designated as holistic attributes, because they appear to characterize the nature of the entire interview, or of large segments of the interview. They may involve verbal and nonverbal behaviors, reflect an attitude or demeanor, characterize the nature of the relationship, or reflect some aspect of the interaction between the participants. Because of the nonspecific nature of these characteristics, their evaluation and the judgment of their presence or absence is accomplished through the use of rating scales. This scale appears on the evaluation forms in Appendix A.

The second category is much more specific and has the characteristic of ostensibility. This category includes observable and quantifiable counseling and interviewing behaviors whose frequency of occurrence can actually be tabulated. These specific counseling behaviors are also listed in the evaluative forms in Appendix A.

The issues of focus, intentionality, trust, attitude, judgmentalness, and feelings and emotions permeate the attributes listed in both the holistic and specific facilitative and nonfacilitative attributes listed in each of the evaluation tables.

The holistic factors may vary and/or provide a general portrait of the interview and counseling session. Their value is in providing a reflection of what is going on between the participants. In all likelihood, they may also vary with the specific interviewing behaviors that are yet to be considered. They certainly can interact with and be influenced by the timing of the counselor changing his or her role to the role of speech/hearing/language therapist.

These associations are highly individualized and vary from problem to problem and even from person to person having the same communication problem.

The vehicle for addressing these issues in a clinical interview starts with a system of tactics for encouraging people to talk to you, to examine themselves and what they feel and believe, which can be factors either in remaining stuck in a problem, or factors in moving forward and progressing through therapy. The skills for how and when to change roles from being the clinician (teacher), with focus on changing speech behavior, and at other times being the counselor, who focuses on beliefs and feelings, could be the difference between overall success or failure in therapy.

The clinical relationship starts to evolve with the first contact between the client and the clinician, developing its style and form, functioning as the client moves through the various behavioral phases of his therapy. It is as though two parallel, interacting processes and experiences go on at the same time, one focusing on the behavioral aspects of changing the way the client talks, and another focusing on such things as feelings, motivation, trust, support, honesty, affection, and respect between the two participants, as the client tries to integrate his new speaking behavior into his life.

We examine what can happen in this clinical relationship, and in turn relate it to the broadly defined phases and processes that focus on speech. Our hope is to develop a sense of the interactions between the focus on speech, and the attributes and processes of the clinical relationship that focuses on the emotional aspects of going through a therapeutic experience.

Although we are describing what appears to be experiences typical of most clients going through therapy for a communication problem, we also are relating material that is highly individualized and sometimes quite atypical. Our comments are based on things that clients have told us during therapy, what they talked about as they changed their speech, their interpretations of themselves, and of course, our own interpretations of their comments and behavior.

As the client begins his therapy, his expectations and beliefs about himself, about his problem, about the program of therapy, and about the clinician, are the most paramount issues. Many of the initial behavioral tactics and strategies of the clinician focus on these issues. Very often, the client enters therapy believing that he cannot rid himself of his problem, and feels quite helpless and victimized. He may believe that there are things going on inside his body or his mind over which he has little control.

These beliefs can be seen across the board, especially in long standing, nonorganic communication problems, whether they be articulation and phonology, voice, fluency, culturally based language differences, or developmental language problems.

These beliefs are also common among the elderly who are going through a number of simultaneous transitions associated with aging, coping with such permanent issues as memory loss, dementia, and linguistic and speaking problems associated with brain damage. Sometimes, the client may think that something happens to him in mysterious and unpredictable ways. These feelings and beliefs can be so strong that the client may not wish to get his hopes too high. He may not feel that he is worth the effort because of past futilities and because he has become convinced that he is inferior in some very basic fiber of his being. He may have a healthy suspicion of therapy and of clinicians. He probably tracks his failures and weaknesses, including the way he talks, rather than his strengths and successes. In his own eyes, he may seem to be a miserable, inadequate, inferior failure as a human being. The possibility of acquiring speech that is free of his problem, and all of the social and emotional implications of that change, are too foreign to even consider and examine. Therefore one of the first and perhaps continuing issues to address during therapy is the client's sense of his own worth, and his development of his "will to recover."

This does not mean that the clinician necessarily delays behavioral strategies that are designed to change his speech until he develops a will to recover or develops a feeling that he is worth changing; rather it means that such behavioral tactics may be exploited for this purpose, and actually facilitate the development of such beliefs. Demonstrations for the client of his control over various elements of his speech mechanism can be relatively easy to arrange, and can become a powerful experiential force in counseling about this issue. Experiencing his own ability to change the way he talks, even briefly, can be especially helpful in shaping the client's expectations and beliefs. Of course, the clinician's interpretations of these brief demonstrations of change and control of speech are also critical to understanding their significance. In addition to Strupp's comments about the importance of trust, Lennard and Bernstein (1960) pointed out that the client must have faith in the clinician as someone who knows what he is doing. Such demonstrations of the counselor/clinician guiding the client into gaining control over his speech mechanism help to reinforce that faith and encourage the client to take the risks involved in turning himself over to the care and nurturing and tactics of the clinician, and ultimately to his own self-control (Kanfer & Karoly 1972).

We have observed clients with communication problems in therapy engaging in the same type of struggle against trusting the clinician, against having faith in the clinician's therapy, and the same type of submission, and the same types of therapeutic bonds of affection that were described by Strupp during psychotherapy. These processes for developing trust may be generally universal for anyone who is vulnerable and forced to go into a "helping relationship" where he is dependent on the "worthiness" and honesty and good will of the clinician. At some stage in therapy, the client starts to believe in the therapy, to trust the clinician, and to submit to the relationship. Trusting the clinician and experiencing change in communication behavior go hand in hand. They feed each other, and are a continuing combined force during all aspects of therapy, but especially in the later stages of social carry over of new skills into the client's everyday world of social interactions.

Whether it be counseling or behavioral conditioning for speech behavior, trust is an important aspect of our work. Just as trust is important to both counseling and to speech therapy, we should also point out that client-centeredness is not restricted to the process of counseling. Client-centeredness could become a process utilized in working on the communication problem as well; and conditioning tactics are not restricted to use in working on communication problems, but can also be employed in counseling tactics.

Ivey (1983) presented what could be considered a powerful rationale for viewing both the process of clinical interviewing as well as the acquisition of interviewing skills within the framework of reinforcement tactics and shaping through successive approximations. He identified a number of specific behaviors (some of which we use in our everyday routines) that can be gradually "shaped" into form, and combined with one another for their deliberate and appropriate use during interviews. Each of these specific behaviors can be operationally defined. Their occurrences can be individually tabulated and counted with relatively minimal error and judgment. Also, there are behaviors, attitudes, and characteristics of large segments of an interview that can be rated in a more holistic perspective as to whether they were helpful or unhelpful or are characteristic of large segments of an interview. All of these are conceptualized as having specific functions that can be used to influence the behavior of the interviewee. In this sense, these specific and holistic interviewing characteristics described by Ivey may function as discriminative stimuli, as positive or negative reinforcers, and as punishers for the responses of the interviewee (Rogers & Skinner, 1956). As we examine each of these specific interviewing behaviors, their functions as events that strengthen, maintain, or weaken the behaviors of the interviewee will be quite apparent. By viewing these events during an interview in both a clinical as well as a conditioning perspective, we add to their understandability, clarify their functions, encourage a sharper and more refined conception of goals for the interviewee, and enable an assessment of their effectiveness as interviewing tactics.

INTEGRATING PERSON-CENTERED THERAPY (ROGERS); MICROCOUNSELING (IVEY); AND OPERANT CONDITIONING (SKINNER)

The literature and background that involves both laboratory studies and less-controlled clinical studies dealing with conditioning during interviews, along with the concepts of micro-units developed by Ivey, the principles of intentionality developed by Authier and Ivey, the principles of Skinner involving various forms of reinforcement, and the principles of Rogers involving client centeredness, self-discovery, and self-actualization as well as experiencing, and the concepts of Rotter involving locus of control, and of Strupp involving trust and affection, are the primary underlying bases for the views we have developed about the clinical interview in Speech Pathology. It is a combination of:

1. The Carl Rogers principles of the "*person-centered approach.*"
2. The B. F. Skinner principles of operant conditioning, which by definition require a focus on contingencies of reinforcement, and a special emphasis on the process of "shaping" through successive approximations.
3. The principles developed by Ivey of microcounseling in interviewing, which by definition require an identification and definition of specific interviewing behaviors, and intentionality by Ivey and Authier, that are facilitative toward certain specific goals for the process of counseling.
4. An awareness and an acknowledgment of the importance of nonspecific factors that may be better conceptualized in less specific, more holistic terms.

The Microcounseling Approach

The microcounseling approach to learning to interview can be seen as involving several related processes:

1. Acquiring specific new behaviors
2. Learning when to practice these behaviors
3. Learning to practice them in combination with one another
4. Learning when to practice behaviors that are already a part of our repertoire at appropriate times during an interview

In operant conditioning terminology, we are talking about:

1. Learning new responses
2. Establishing stimulus control over new and old, previously learned responses.

These latter terms come from the operant experimental laboratory and imply a precision of control over the conditions that prevail that may be only minimally possible during an interview. However, these terms do offer the principles that guide our task of learning interviewing skills. Things happen rapidly during an interview, the stimuli from the participants are numerous and varied in form, and the control over what happens is shared among the participants. We should acknowledge that instating specific behaviors and establishing stimulus control over their emission as practiced in the laboratory is a far cry from applying these principles and tactics to training in interviewing skills. It serves, however, as an important guide for the process of intentionality in acquiring these skills. Once we have acquired experience in deliberately using these separate behaviors, one at a time and in small combinations, many of them will become more or less automatic and we will not have to think about them. We may find that we will be gradually reinforced over time by our clients for certain behaviors, and this may establish our interviewing style. However, some of the behaviors may never become automatic, but will always require deliberation and forethought.

A special notation should be made of the thinking of Ivey and Authier regarding the idea that learning to interview requires a process of "learning by doing." This idea was translated into a system of "Learning by Doing" practice projects that is employed throughout this book. The learning of each of the interviewing behaviors involves actually engaging in that behavior, doing it in a practice project, with an interviewing partner, until it is established as part of your repertoire. This same learning by doing practicing tactic is used later for gradually layering these separate behaviors, one into the other, until they become integrated into a style of communication that takes on the attributes of the thoughts, beliefs, attitudes, vocabulary, and actions that are appropriate for a clinical interview.

Before we consider the specific interviewing behaviors, let us first consider how we as clinicians can help establish the kind of clinical relationship that will interact with and facilitate our speech conditioning program.

Recognizing the many emotional parameters of a human being in distress, and the individual feelings of clients as they enter and progress through speech therapy, we see that as clinicians we have several functions. We are at the same time teachers and counselors, and although we may be able to keep a clear view of when we are doing what, it might not be that clear to our clients. One moment we may be the authority figure providing all kinds of technical information, and the next moment asking our client "What do you think is going on?"

A good rule of thumb that could function as a reminder for us is: "We are generally functioning as teachers when we establish the agenda for what is happening. We are functioning as counselors when we encourage the client to establish the agenda."

The talking that goes on between the clinician and the client, even when the clinician is functioning as a counselor, is providing the client with real life opportunities for practicing his new speech skills. This talking time is critically important practice time for the client in transferring his skills from protected to less-protected talking environments.

We are functioning as counselors when we minimize our influence on the content of what is being talked about, when we encourage the client's efforts to set the content agenda, and when we facilitate the client's efforts to look at himself and his emotional reactions to the experiences he is encountering as he changes the way he talks and the way he feels about himself. Of course, when the content seems to wander into irrelevance, or when a content area has been overlooked that you the counselor, think is important, then it is appropriate to bring the client gently around to addressing that content. But everything doesn't have to be addressed in the first interview, and in fact it may be more helpful at times to delay discussing certain content, until a strong and trusting relationship has developed between the client and the clinician.

Getting the therapeutic-conditioning process started depends on the ability of the clinician to help the client talk to him. His skills as an interviewer become paramount in helping the client move through the various phases of therapy.

The clinician as a skilled interviewer therefore addresses two important processes in therapy. One of these is to provide the client with opportunities to accumulate large amounts of talking time for gaining experience with his new talking skills. The second process is that, as a skilled interviewer, he facilitates the client's trust, love, sense of worth, self-understanding, and insight, as well as his personal responsibility for solving his own problems.

Our role is to facilitate the client's self-explorations and verbal expressions; to help him examine his thoughts and feelings about important issues as he enters into and progresses through therapy. In the beginning, because of his history, he may dwell on his particular problem, and on his historical, social and emotional investments in his problem. Or, as he experiences changes in his speech with his clinician, he may examine his fears, doubts, and expectations for the future—his future as a former speech defective. Whatever the content may be, it is established by the client. Our job is to focus on the client, helping him to see that he is the focus and that we are there to facilitate his experience.

6

LISTENING AND ATTENDING

The holistic property of listening and attending is a factor in all of the behaviors and attributes to be discussed. It is the basic building block for the counselor's focus on the client and the counselor's intentionality. Intentionality refers to the counselor's purposeful control over his own behaviors. It underlies all of the facilitative specific and holistic factors you will be considering in your analyses of your interviews. The counselor's attention and listening is revealed by his body language and posture, his gaze patterns, his verbal comments that directly relate to what the client has just said, and by his sensitivity and warmth and acceptance throughout the interview. Without listening and attending the rest of it doesn't happen.

To be listened to by someone is one of the highest compliments an individual may experience. Close listening and sustained attending by the counselor is one of his most powerful reinforcers for talkativeness. Take it away and the client's talkativenss can disappear.

Furthermore, selective attending by the counselor encourages the client to focus on specific aspects of what he has been talking about. Again, without very close selective attending by the counselor to such things as emotional expressions, or the circumstances for emotional expressions, such focus by the client will not occur. This particular holistic attribute is the backbone of counseling, it makes it all happen, like the starter and gas pump on an automobile. The counselor's interest, attitude, warmth, and valuing of the client develop from and is communicated to the client by the counselor's listening and attending behaviors.

Close listening and attending on the surface seems like a fairly simple and uncomplicated thing to do. It is certainly learnable. But at the same time, over the typical period of a 1-hour counseling interview, we should realize in advance that listening and attending is an exhausting transaction. The counselor subordinates himself, his ideas, his needs, and all other thoughts about his life outside of this session, and gives complete attention to the client. He hangs onto the client's every word and action. He should be able to receive, store, and retrieve what the client says to him, put that client's feelings into words and store that as well. He may also interpret, sometimes if only to himself, the meaning and understandings he develops from the client's revelations.

This tactic of listening and attending evolves into a complicated process for several reasons. It is an exhausting effort to sustain a focus on "the words," that is, the auditory, phonic stimulus to one's hearing mechanism, and to be able to store and retrieve those words. Added to this is the need to become selective within that focus on the words, and the need to also keep track of the content of those words, and to decipher their meanings, as well as being aware of yourself and your own reactions, and being able to subordinate yourself and your reactions.

Several important processes are going on within the counselor almost simultaneously and it takes great concentration and effort by the counselor both to engage in it, and to communicate to the client that it is going on.

It is important for the client to realize that he is being closely attended to because it tells him that he is valued by the counselor, and therefore he also may begin to value himself.

SUGGESTED PRACTICE PROJECTS

All of the behaviors to be discussed and learned involve and imply close attending and listening. Therefore these several practicing exercises may be considered the building blocks and foundations for the more sophisticated and actual counseling behaviors.

The initial goal, for practice purposes, outside of the context of the interview, is listening—to extend our listening skills to their limits.

To actually practice these skills will require a little preparation that will enable the practice itself to move more rapidly and effectively.

This is an initial exercise in listening. You want to find out how far you can push your listening behavior, how much you can hear, store, and retrieve, moving from very simple to longer and more meaningful material.

This will involve two people working together, and changing roles. One person will function as the "feeder" and one as the "receiver."

The task is for the receiver to repeat, verbatim, what the feeder says or reads to him.

The task starts out easy. The feeder says one word such as "well." The receiver repeats that word. Then the feeder says the word "yes" and the receiver repeats that word. The feeder is sending out "one-word" messages that have no relationship to each other. When the receiver can repeat, verbatim, each one-word message three times, the feeder increases the message to a two-word unit. For example "were-but." When the receiver can repeat three of these two-word units correctly, consecutively, the feeder increases it to a four-word unit. The feeder has to be able to keep track of the number of words he is uttering each time. He can probably handle this mentally, up to four-word units. After four-word units, we have found that it makes sense to mark up a magazine, newspaper, or journal article in advance to keep accurate track of the feeder's task. The example given is a marked-up text from some material in a book. The slash mark indicates the boundaries of that particular word unit, and is immediately punctuated by the feeder pausing to hear the receiver's echoing response. The goal is to get three units in a row correct before increasing the unit by one word. If the receiver gets one word wrong in trying to get three in a row, the feeder starts that unit over again at the beginning of the next sentence. This is continued until the receiver gets three in a row correct, or three in a row incorrect, consecutively. This is considered the receiver's limit for that day. This can be done several times in an attempt to increase such close listening as much as possible. Of necessity, it requires a form of invoking self-discipline and control to execute a particular behavior and reinforces the focus and intentionality of the counselor's behavior.

Practice Text

One-Word Unit:

> "The"/ (feeder pauses for receiver's echoing response), /"goals"/ (feeder pauses for receiver's echoing response), /"of"/
>
> "science"/"are"/"to"/"explain"/"predict"/"and"/"control"
>
> /"events"/"in"/"nature"/

Two-Word Unit:

> "Most areas/of speech/language pathology/are still/ largely involved/in the/description of/the signs/and symptoms"/

Three-Word Unit:

> "Such is the/case for stuttering/Stuttering is a/disability of spoken/ language that emerges/most often at/a time when"/

Four-Word Unit:

"From biblical times to/ the present stuttering has/defied explanation. What it/is and where it"/

Five-Word Unit:

"Recently however advances in genetics/in particular genetic engineering have/focused some researchers on the/was the role of theory"/

Six-Word Unit:

"What is the theory and why/do we devote so much time/a theory provides a statement of"/

Seven-Word Unit:

"In such a situation would you sit/down with the animal and take a/ the classic nature versus nurture controversy had"/

Eight-Word Unit:

"Perhaps however the most important reason to investigate/etiology is that if we identify the origins/his theory offers both an explanation of how"/

Nine-Word Unit:

"If he was correct in stating that the young/children become developmentally disfluent their preschool years the significance/so many youngsters having their behavioral repertoires speech patterns"/

Ten-Word Unit:

"Given these difficulties there is yet value in exploring the/etiology of stuttering. The theory focused on normal speech development/strategy was truly correct in pursuing the need for counseling"/

Eleven-Word Unit:

"An alternative etiological approach would be to observe the dynamics of/neither of these kinds of data comes out of experimental studies/ This publication became the thesis for most of the content and"/

Twelve-Word Unit:

> "Although a substantial amount of information has been accumulated about childhood stuttering/and a number of promising leads have been uncovered, conclusive evidence is/not yet available to implicate any of these leads as contributing factors."/

A reasonable and functional goal is to be able to echo, verbatim, a 10- to 15-word unit, three consecutive times.

The next project in the progression of listening and attending is for the feeder to engage in a mock interview, wherein he or she will pause after each phrase or utterance to enable the receiver (interviewer) to again echo, verbatim, that immediately preceding phrase or utterance. Typically, most utterances are no longer than about 10 to 12 words, and therefore such an exercise begins to approximate what might be encountered in a real interview. Again, the criterion of three consecutive phrases repeated correctly should be used before moving on to a more natural condition.

The next project is the same as the previous one, except that the feeder does not have to pause after each utterance or phrase, and the receiver attempts to repeat as much as he can of what he has heard.

It is quite unlikely that long, verbatim echoing by the interviewer of a client's entire verbal response will take place very often during an actual interview.

These listening exercises have been deliberately exaggerated to give the interviewer the experience of very close attending beyond what is necessary, as well as to enhance his focus and intentionality.

At this point, your practicing of attending has prepared you to move on into the learning of actual specific behaviors that have application to real-life counseling situations.

7

SPECIFIC FACILITATIVE INTERVIEWING BEHAVIORS

Ivey and Authier (1978) designate four major clusters of interviewing skills: (a) beginning skills; (b) selective listening skills; (c) self-expression skills; and (d) interpretation skills. The four titles of these clusters do not refer to the behaviors themselves but, rather, suggest their functions or timing or uniqueness. Within these clusters are 13 specific behaviors that occupy most of our attention. All of these specific facilitative interviewing behaviors are listed in Table A.1 in Appendix A.

According to Ivey, the beginning skills in interviewing have two basic functions: to assist the client in talking and expressing himself, and to give the novice interviewer a feeling of success, confidence, and something specific to fall back on if he or she gets confused or loses focus during the interview. However, it should be pointed out that these behaviors may also contribute to the trust and affection that a client may develop as he or she experiences the prizing and respect that the clinician shows for him or her and his or her problems.

There are three behaviors to consider in this beginning phase of learning to interview. These are:

1. Attending behavior
2. Open-invitations to talk
3. Minimal encouragers to talk

ATTENDING BEHAVIORS

Silent Listening

Interviewing is an active process of both listening and talking by all participants. Listening is as active a process as talking. Listening is a part of the clinician's general attending behavior that involves both verbal and nonverbal activity. Being naturally attentive, relaxed, and maintaining good contact verbally and nonverbally with the client will permit him to talk comfortably about what he wants, in his own way. The clinician should let this happen without getting in the way or impeding such a process. This close attention via silent listening by the clinician can communicate several things to the client:

1. If the clinician closely listens to him, the client can develop a stronger sense of valuing himself. Close listening by the counselor can communicate to the client that what he has to say is worth attending to. This effort on the part of the clinician is easily perceived by the client and translates into a feeling that the clinician is willing to put forth such an effort, and thus respects and values the client. Such a perception can enhance the client's feelings of self-worth.
2. Such close silent listening can help the client see the clinician as one who is genuinely concerned about him and that he is really there and available to be of help.
3. Through such listening, the focus of the sessions begins to take shape and the roles of each participant become more sharply defined. The client begins to develop a sense of his own responsibility, as well as a sense of the clinician's responsibilities during the therapeutic interviews. He will become comfortable with how the clinician accepts him and does not judge him and as a result will begin to take those first risky steps of personal revelation, sharing, and trust.

It is essential that the attending behavior by the counselor permits the client to establish his own agenda of content, in his own time, through his own defenses and resistances and in his own style. The role of the counselor (speech clinician) is to let this happen and to facilitate the process. Behaviorists might add, as another way to understand what is going on between the counselor and the client, "The counselor is reinforcing the talkativeness of the client."

Many important and positive things may be communicated to the client as he goes through this process of getting started and of being attended to, both from the client to himself as well as from the clinician.

SUGGESTED PRACTICE PROJECT

With your classmate or short-term practice partner you can practice silent listening during a few minutes of a mock interview. After an open invitation to talk, such as "Tell me what your day has been like," the "counselor" in this practice project should try to limit himself to "silent listening." You should do this while maintaining good eye contact and other nonverbal attending behaviors. Push yourself beyond your own "silent comfort level," just for the experience of it, and to see what the effect is on your short-term interviewing partner.

Verbal Following

As the client starts off on his "journey into self," as Rogers (1942) termed it, he begins to feel that he will be shouldering the responsibility for identifying and exploring and expressing the nature of those things that are of significance for him. He will begin to recognize his own defensive devices and methods for protecting himself, from himself, and from the clinician, as well as how he, the client, interferes with himself.

Besides active, silent listening, the most specific and identifiable aspects of attending behavior involve "verbally following" the content of what the client is talking about. It involves closely tracking what the client is saying so that the content can be accurately stored, retrieved, and reflected back to the client. Comments and questions by the clinician should relate directly to what the client has said to him. Such verbal following can also communicate and stress the respect that the clinician has for the client's content and ideas and feelings, as well as style and language, that characterize the issues he is considering important at that moment. Such verbal following and echoing of the client can function as an encouragement to the client to continue what he was talking about. Sometimes, merely repeating the last word or two uttered by the client has a powerful effect on the client's continued verbalizing. Your goal for "listening and verbal following" is to learn to repeat as exactly and as accurately as possible what might be said to you. Such accuracy in listening and repeating will ultimately maximize the interviewer's ability to store and retrieve and express the verbal material presented by a client. It reduces the clinician's errors in reproducing that material or selective portions of that material because he bypasses his own subjective filtering by disciplining himself to stay with the language of the client.

SUGGESTED PRACTICE PROJECT

Meet again with your short-term interviewing partner, for a short 5-minute interview. After issuing an open invitation to talk, the "counselor" should limit himself to echoing only the last two or three words uttered by the short-term interviewing partner. Even though the partner knows that what is going on is a practice maneuver, he will usually succumb to the "reinforcing" properties of this type of minimal encouragement (echoing and verbal following), and continue talking.

Nonverbal Communication

Appropriate eye contact, posture, physical distance and space, and body movement are all a part of the array of nonverbal elements that communicate that the client is being closely attended. The client will gradually get comfortable with the idea and the experience of sharing his innermost, private self with another human being. WHY? Because he, the client, and perhaps all of us on occasion need to be closely attended to by another human being—and the clinician is there to provide it.

The practice of these nonverbal elements of communication should be a part of all of the counseling practice projects you engage in.

OPEN INVITATION TO TALK

During the interview the clinician can provide the client with open invitations to talk. Such invitations give the client a maximum opportunity to talk, and to compose his content with minimal influences by the clinician. The source of significant information is the client, as he sees it, thinks it, feels it, verbalizes it, and defends against it. The length, complexity, and themes of what the client communicates are determined by the client.

The "open invitation" communicates the clinician's respect for these issues and his desire for the client to take those first risky steps of personal revelation. It also minimizes presumptions by the clinician about what may or may not be important for the client to explore and talk about.

Very often open invitations to talk take the form of an instruction or an open-ended question from the clinician such as:

Open Instructions
1. "Tell me why you came here today."
2. "Tell me about your family."

Open Questions
1. "What was it like, living on a boat?"
2. "What did you feel at the time she told you this?"

SUGGESTED PRACTICE PROJECTS

With a classmate or with your short-term interviewing partner, conduct a short interview wherein you limit your verbalizing to open invitations to talk. You can vary these between "open questions" and "open instructions." When your partner pauses, or has completed his response, insert another open invitation for him to respond but try to keep it related to what he has just talked about. After doing this for 5 minutes, reverse roles. After each partner has had an opportunity to practice the "open invitations," try an additional 5 minutes by adding your "echoing" of the last two or three words uttered by your partner before issuing your "open invitation." You can now continue your interview for another 5 minutes using your "silent listening," your "verbal following," and your "open invitations."

These behaviors should now deliberately be tried out in your interviews with your long-term interviewing partner.

Closed Invitations to Talk

Closed interview formats are easily differentiated from open structures. For example:

1. "Are you married?"
2. "What is your spouse's name, age, and occupation?"
3. "Did you live on a boat or in a house?"

Such a closed approach usually limits the responsiveness of the client to a few words, or a mere affirmation or denial of material composed by the clinician. The closed question or closed instruction may have some valuable functions during an interview, when delimiting areas of content is appropriate. The theme is determined by the clinician. However, there can be instances when the interviewer believes he provided an open structure and it functions as a closed one, or has provided a closed structure and it operates like an open one. The following are some additional examples, including the client's responses:

Clinician's Stimulus	*Client's Response*	*Stim./Resp. Function*
1. "Did you have any trouble today?"	"yes"	close/close
2. "Do you get embarrassed?"	"yes"	close/close
3. "What's your name?"	"John Doe"	close/close
4. "Your address?"	"I moved three times last year"	close/open
5. "Do you live at home?"	"Not now. I did for 10 years."	close/open
6. "How did it happen?"	"Who knows?"	open/close

Closed structures obviously have their functions during interviews, when denial or affirmation are sought, or when specific identifying information is required. They are also valuable when used in combination with open structures. For example:

Clinician's Stimulus	Client's Response
1. "Are you married?" (closed)	"yes"
2. "How did you meet your wife?" (open)	"We met at a party." (content is composed)
3. "Do you have any children?" (closed)	"yes"
4. "Tell me about them." (open)	"I have 3 boys, teenagers"(content is composed)

However, we should be careful, and it is a common occurrence, not to shut off an open invitation to talk by following it too rapidly with a closed question. For example: The clinician asks, "What was it like, living on a boat?" (open) "I mean, did you sleep on a bed or a bunk?" (closed)

Although we should be very careful about proposing any axioms of absolute "dos and don'ts," in interviewing, we would like to alert you to be cautious about how a question is worded, so that you *do not* communicate a desired answer as you pose the question. For example, a series of questions might illustrate this point:

1. "How old are you?"
2. "And do you still live with your parents?"
3. "Have you thought of being on your own?"

The latter two questions in the series contain words and ideas that probably communicate some value judgments and socially desirable and undesirable responses. Perhaps a better approach to this information, if it is at all deemed pertinent, would be:

1. "Tell me about where you live."
2. "Tell me about your family."
3. "How long have you lived where you are now?"
4. "Any plans for making a change?"

These are all possibilities that minimize the probability of telling the client that you want to hear a particular type of acceptable content in his response.

SUGGESTED PRACTICE PROJECTS

With your classmate or short-term interviewing partner, conduct an interview for 5 minutes where you limit the interviewer's behavior to asking only closed questions. As soon as the partner pauses, insert another closed question. Observe the effect on the interviewee. It will probably involve very brief answers with little clarification.

After taking turns at doing this exercise, practice asking closed questions that lead into "open questions" for another 2 minutes, just to get the feel of how the "closed–open" tandem can be productive in first getting the interviewee into a particular content area, and then giving him the freedom to compose what he wants to tell you.

MINIMAL ENCOURAGERS TO TALK

Like the open invitation to talk, this interviewing tactic also involves minimal influences by the clinician. It is usually employed after the client has started talking, and is designed to keep him talking, if that is the clinician's wish, without interrupting him. It may be nonverbal, such as a periodic nodding of the head; it may also be verbal, such as saying:

"Could you explain that more?"

"I see."

"I understand."

"Hum hm . . ."

"Yes!"

"Uh-huh . . ."

"I don't quite understand."

"Tell me more about that."

Other tactics include:

Silence and maintaining eye contact.

Repeating the last few words of the client's comment.

Offering an incomplete phrase for the client to pick up on, for example," And then," "And after that," "And then you said. . . ."

These behaviors are relatively easy to acquire and become almost automatic with experience. One of the more critical aspects of this behavior, however, is for the interviewer to get control of its emission, to make sure that he employs it when he wants to, and inhibits it when it is not appropriate. It should be noted that general attending devices and minimal encouragers to talk can function as positive reinforcers for the client's talkativeness as well as for specific content areas. However, if such behaviors become too automatic or are used without thought by the clinician, the clinician could easily find himself attending and listening and encouraging material that he feels may not be pertinent to the therapy. There may be times when the clinician may not want to strengthen or maintain the particular content being explored or expressed by the client, yet the client may continue to talk about these same things, possibly because the clinician is inadvertently reinforcing such content with his minimal encouragers. They easily can become too automatic as general attending devices, and therefore function as a reinforcer for specific, but undesirable content. The clinician must sort out these functions of minimal encouragers for the client to talk and be able to use each of them appropriately.

SUGGESTED PRACTICE PROJECTS

An interesting training exercise for acquiring this type of behavior (minimal encouragers to talk) is to deliberately use it, exclusively, without resorting to questions and other invitations to talk, for short segments of a practice interview. Even when interviewees are aware of the tactics being employed, the interviewer's behavior functions as a positive reinforcer for the interviewee's responsiveness, sometimes to the amazement of both participants. After engaging in this practice interview for 5 minutes, then conduct another 10-minute practice interview using all of the behaviors you have been practicing, including the minimal encouragers. Again, these minimal encouragers should be deliberately used in your interview with your long-term interviewing partner, when they seem to be appropriate.

SELECTIVE ATTENTION

Emerging from the beginning skills of interviewing, which may be characterized as interviewing behaviors that generally reinforce "talkativeness" by a client, is the need to develop the purpose and focus of the interviews. Certain aspects of the things that the client talks about may be deemed more pertinent to his problems than others. We are therefore in a position to selectively reinforce those more pertinent aspects. The first step in such differential reinforcement is to designate the various forms of responses by the client that we may wish to strengthen, maintain, or weaken.

Rogers (1942, 1972) and Seeman (1986) have dichotomized client's responses in terms of "emotions or feelings" as opposed to "cognition and reasoning."

We refer to this same dichotomy as "expressions of feelings," that may be differentiated from "content that describes the circumstances for those feelings." However, sometimes the person's feelings become the circumstances for additional feelings. For example, examine the statement, "She lied to me" (the circumstance), "and I felt angry" (the feeling), "and I enjoyed being angry at her. Then I felt guilty." There are feelings of anger that become the circumstance for feeling enjoyment, which in turn become the circumstance for feeling guilty.

There is also a difference between past feelings and current feelings. In the earlier example we had a description of a past feeling. If the clinician had noted from the client's tone of voice, rate of speech, or other verbal and nonverbal cues, other feelings that were in the here and now of relating the past, these could also be designated as responses for some type of differential reinforcement or action by the clinician. We may want to weaken the past feelings while strengthening the current feelings. In any event, we must have a rationale for what we select to strengthen, maintain, or weaken.

The more general rationale for selectively responding to a client's feelings is that *people behave and act on the basis of what they believe and feel.*

If you reject that general rationale, then there will be little need to reinforce the expression of past and/or current feelings. However, more specifically, we may see in individual clients that their feelings and beliefs relate directly to their communication problem, either as a cue that triggers the occurrence, as a maintaining consequent factor, or as something that is generated by their communication problem. We may also hypothesize that the client's feelings are leading him to behave in ways that interfere with his functioning, such as in self-pity, anger, depression, and helplessness. If we view communication problems as involving the complexities of the total human experience and condition, then it becomes clear that the way a person feels about himself, about others, about his speech as a part of himself, and about changing himself, is as much a part of our concern as the tactics we employ to instate new motor talking behavior.

Paraphrasing Content

Selective attention by the interviewer implies that the interviewer has decided to pay attention to a particular aspect of the verbal material being presented to him. One of these aspects can be the cognitive content, or situations, or circumstances about which the client is talking. However, such selective attending by the interviewer to these circumstances is really designed to encourage the client to attend to such material. Open and closed questions as well as minimal encouragers that directly relate to such material can function to direct the client's attention to these circumstances, such as,

1. "Tell me about your family." (open invitation)
2. "Are your parents here in the city?" (closed question)
3. "What is it like to live in the same area as your parents?" (open question)

4. "I'm not sure I understand what you said about your parents." (minimal encourager)

Another interviewing tactic that can function in a similar fashion is to have the counselor paraphrase the material that the client just told him. This means putting the material into your own words and saying it back to the client. The counselor in a sense functions to mirror the material back to the client, so that the client hears his own message. He can then amplify, clarify, correct, revise, or confirm. If there are confusions or double messages, such feedback will more sharply define their existence and call for clarification. In this way, the client can get in touch with himself and his thoughts because they have been reproduced in an instant replay for him. There may be times during an interview when it is appropriate to probe deeply into a particular circumstance (e.g., goals, sex, religion, family, education, etc.). The counselor may wish to encourage the client to talk more about a subject in order to promote mutual understanding of his role in it, or because that particular topic appears to be at the core of the client's problems. Paraphrasing the client's utterances of the content of a particular topic can help to bring about that mutual understanding.

However, there is an additional value to the tactic of paraphrasing content. By encouraging the client to describe, to clarify, and to amplify, very often the client may recreate and re-experience certain aspects of what he is describing. In some instances, actual past dialogues and conversations are reproduced in the here and now of the client. This recreation of a situation, or thinking through of an experience, may also recreate earlier feelings and emotions associated with the experience or generate new and current feelings about the material. Therefore we may be able to encourage the expressions of feelings by the client by focusing on the descriptive details of the circumstance or situation, and it may help the participants get in touch with some emotional material that might otherwise remain hidden and unavailable.

One becomes skillful in doing these things, by doing them; by practicing them with an interviewing partner so that eventually, even within the context of a client-centered interview, the counselor can influence the process.

Pennebaker in his book *Opening Up* (1990) wrote about the healing power of confiding in others. He stated that inhibition takes much work, and activates stressors in the body that can lead to physical illness. It should be noted that inhibition is one of the major self-administered consequences of living with a communication problem, and the processes of counseling that we have been addressing is a major attempt to alleviate such stress and eliminate these tendencies to inhibit speaking and to avoid talking situations.

SUGGESTED PRACTICE PROJECTS

The vehicle for practicing "paraphrasing of content" can take many forms. One is with your classmate or short-term interviewing partner, wherein you engage in the usual invitations to talk to get your partner talking to you, but then when he pauses, you deliberately limit yourself to putting that material into your own words, and saying it back to him. Do not use his language, use your own composition of the material.

In addition to this, you can get much more practice by merely listening to the TV news, and putting the commentator's message into your own words, or doing the same in some of your everyday conversations with friends. It should be intentional and deliberate when you do it, so that you sense your control over your own verbal behavior.

Summarizing Content

Unlike paraphrasing content, whose referent is the immediately preceding utterance by the client, "summarizing" the client's content involves paraphrasing longer segments of the client's output, perhaps 10 or 15 minutes of material. It does not involve a verbatim repetition of the client's utterances, but rather a succinct but accurate recounting and feedback. However, there may be some crucial judgments made by the counselor of what to include and what not to include in a summary statement. Usually the counselor is trying to grasp "the big message" and will ignore what he considers unimportant. He will give feedback only on the most significant material. Such judgments can easily be in error, but usually the client will correct such errors of either omission or commission.

Summarization of content during an interview can function in several ways. During a series of interviews it can be an effective method for initiating a particular session:

> Counselor: "The last time we were together you were telling me that you were seriously thinking of taking a new job in another city."

Summarization can also be useful to determine whether the client has gone as far as he wishes to go in exploring a particular subject area:

> Counselor: "I think I understand. You want to think some more about changing your job and the implications of that change."

Summarization can be combined with a minimal encourager to enhance further exploration by the client:

Counselor: "The message I've been getting here is that you're thinking of moving to another city and changing jobs. Is this a major issue for you now, or . . . ?"

Summarization can also be used at the end of a particular interview to more or less clarify what has gone on during a session:

Counselor: "We've really talked about a lot of different things today, but somehow we always come back to the issue of changing jobs and moving."

Finally, summarization can be employed to relate areas of concern that otherwise may be perceived as discrete or separate from one another:

Counselor: "We've really talked about a lot of different things today, your friends, your family, your comfort with the city, and the possibility of moving. Do you think they relate to one another in some way?"

SUGGESTED PRACTICE PROJECTS

Summarization of content again involves focusing on the content or circumstance that is being discussed (rather than the feelings associated with that circumstance), and feeding back a succinct summary of the most important points of a large segment of the interview. It does not mean that you function as a tape recorder, feeding back each idea, but instead, sifting through and identifying the most significant aspects of the material. You can practice this in your mock interviews by starting the interview out with a summary of the material covered during your last interview with that person, by closing an interview with a summary, or by inserting a summary during the interview and asking for some clarification. The summary should not be so long or wordy that you are taking up a lot of the interview time with it. A good way to practice the succinctness of it is to do one summary, then immediately make it shorter, in a second attempt. Then make it even shorter in a third attempt. You may be surprised at how succinct you can become with such practice. Each of these should be deliberately carried out during your mock interview, until you feel comfortable with the process and to enable you to experience the effects that it has on your interviewee's behavior.

REFLECTING FEELINGS

The current here and now feelings and emotional expressions of a client may be one of the more difficult processes to facilitate during an interview. Very often a client may try to hide or edit his true feelings about an issue from the counselor as well as from himself. Sometimes his resistances to emotional expressions are in the forms of mechanisms of which even he is unaware.

He may unconsciously refuse to admit his feelings, or he may explain his problem away to avoid his feelings, or engage in some competing activity to escape from his feelings, or even state that others feel something, but he doesn't. He may also consciously resist revealing his feelings because he doesn't trust how the counselor may judge him.

Very often the client seeks approval from the counselor and tries to determine if approval will be forthcoming even before he risks any personal revelations. Skinner has pointed out that "approval" can function as a powerful reinforcer. Yet the counselor, in his desire to create a judgment-free atmosphere, so that the client will explore his innermost and private self, may wish to minimize "approval." The counselor must walk a very tight and narrow line. His comments and behavior should communicate approval, acceptance, and positive judgments of "the process of emotional expression," thereby reinforcing such comments by the client. However, he does not usually wish to judge the validity, appropriateness, or goodness or badness of any one specific or particular emotional expression, even though the client may seek specific approval from the counselor for a specific bit of emotional material. What the client receives from the counselor is acceptance of his expressions of emotional material, not a positive or negative judgment of the content of that material. This appears to be a paradox wherein the client wants something that the counselor cannot give in the form that the client desires. But it may not be as paradoxical as it seems. Perhaps an example will clarify:

> Client: "I was so angry and hurt that I just wanted to be alone, to scream. My own self-pity was disgusting to me. What do you think? Am I crazy or something? Maybe I'm just seeing my point of view. Am I being reasonable in what I feel?"

In this commentary, the client on the surface is asking the counselor to judge him—to judge the appropriateness of his feelings. The counselor could pick up on many things in this client's comments. However, the basic issue is not the validity of the appropriateness of the client's emotions. The counselor's job is to communicate to the client that all of his feelings are valid and appropriate to the client's needs at that time. They happened, they existed, and a judgment of their appropriateness does not erase the history of their occurrence. No amount of intellectualization about them will invalidate them. The counselor accepts their expression, accepts their validity, and moves on from there to determine their functions and influences, to help the client to clarify and amplify and perhaps determine whether these feelings influence his behavior now, whether and how he acts on them, whether they interfere or facilitate his personal growth and understanding, and to determine the motives behind and the consequences of such feelings.

The counselor does not give these understandings to the client, but rather picks up on significant material that has been presented and feeds it back for the client to generate his own understandings. When the counselor reflects a client's feelings back to him, he is trying to get the client to focus on how he feels, to recognize how he feels, to accept the fact that he does indeed feel something about what he is talking about, perhaps to label that feeling and put it into words, and accept it as a part of himself. In addition, he is being urged to explore those feelings, when they occur, the circumstances that are the occasions for their expression, and what form of expression they take. In addition, coming out of this exploration should be an awareness of the consequences of these feelings, and how he acts or behaves as a result of these feelings. This is an important part of self-actualization, wherein the client becomes aware of himself and the forces that drive him to feel, believe, and act in ways that may be helpful or destructive to himself and to others who are important to him, and eventually to making appropriate changes on the basis of this new self-awareness.

In some instances where the relationship between client and counselor has grown to be deep and trusting and where the counselor understands the values of the client, the counselor may occasionally provide a veiled and cautious judgment that reflects the value system of the client, the resistance of the client, or the functions of the client's feelings. However, most often the tactic employed by the counselor is that of reflecting the client's feelings back to him as he perceives them from the specific words uttered, the nonverbal behavior, and the paralinguistic attributes of the client's speech (rate, loudness, inflection, etc.). This process of reflecting feelings requires the counselor to see through, around, and under the surface of the material presented by the client. Very often the client may say one thing but really mean something else. The counselor must understand and interpret for himself the latent meanings and messages from the overt, surface material. He must recognize recurring patterns of resistance mechanisms (e.g., denial, rationalizing, etc.) and how they function to impede getting in touch with latent material.

In the previous example, the surface message was a request for a judgment and for acceptance. However, if we dissect that message further, we may see that the very fact that the question is being asked may mean that the client is judging or has judged himself, and is asking the counselor for a reaffirmation of his acceptance and for an opportunity to explore and understand that part of himself that may not be acceptable, perhaps to rejudge and to re-evaluate and to accept or to reject some aspect of himself further (e.g., "my own self-pity was disgusting to me"). A self-judgment and self-acceptance is not the same as an externally imposed judgment or acceptance by others. But such external acceptances can be helpful to the client as he continues his self-exploration. The counselor may in fact wish to reinforce what is known as an "internal locus of control" rather than an "external locus of control," whereby the client becomes more responsive to his own judgments than to the judgments of others. This client may have felt that a vehicle for self-re-judgment and evaluation was having available the counselor's judgments and acceptance. But the counselor must help the client proceed, with his support, toward independent self-evaluation and re-evaluation and ultimately to independently derived self-understanding and responsibility for his behavior and feelings.

One possible response by the counselor might be:

> Counselor: "You sound like you were very angry at yourself for the way you were feeling, but now with the questions you just asked me, it seems that you're re-evaluating, not only that anger at that time at yourself, but also perhaps that maybe those feelings you had toward her were OK."
>
> "You're already there, you don't need me to tell you."

The specific counseling tactic of "reflecting feelings" requires that the counselor differentiate the emotional material from the cognitive content or circumstance for the emotional expression. The counselor then attempts to label that feeling and to put it into words for the client to respond to.

A few examples may illustrate the process:

1. Client: "I was alone, watching the sunset, yet I didn't feel lonely. It was a beautiful moment. It was all so peaceful."
   Counselor: "You were really moved." (reflection of feeling)
   "by your alone-time, and in touch with yourself."
   (paraphrasing content—an optional response)
2. Client: "When I came in the door my little boy just grinned at me and leaned against me, wanting physical contact. I could see his total, unqualified love, even without any words being said."
   Counselor: "You felt close, very close.
   (reflection of feeling)
   "at that moment to your son."
   (paraphrasing content—optional)
3. Client: "There are still a lot of things that I've kept from you. Personal things that are difficult and painful to look at."
   Counselor: "You sound like you are afraid."

(reflection of feeling)
"to talk about these things."
(paraphrasing content—optional)

To learn this process of reflecting feeling, you have to become facile with the language of feelings. Often the feelings you perceive are expressed nonverbally. Also, the client does not necessarily use feeling words or feeling vocabulary when he lets you see what he is feeling. Yet your job is to communicate back to the client verbally—in words—what you perceive his feelings to be. This means you need to learn the vocabulary for translating the client's feelings into words that you can use to provide feedback to your client.

SUGGESTED PRACTICE PROJECTS

The following is a description of a special project that has proven to be helpful for learning how to identify and reflect affective, emotional responses.

Turn to Appendix B, *Words to Describe Feelings.*

Because it is often difficult to translate emotions and feelings into words, you have been supplied with a list of words that denote specific feelings and emotional states. You should try to learn the formal definition of as many of these terms as possible.

Additionally, with your short-term interviewing partner or a classmate you should engage in the following practice exercise. Compose and utter a statement to your interviewing partner that you think would enable him to recognize a particular feeling that is on that list, but without saying that particular "feeling" word.

For example, if you said, "I was dodging traffic, ducking back and forth between cars, trying to get across the street, when suddenly two cars were coming at me from opposite directions. I moved forward, then backward, then I froze." From the context and language, from the tone of your voice, from how loud or how fast you spoke, your partner might be able to recognize and tell you that the feeling was one of "fear" or "fright," even though those words were never used by the speaker. Do this exercise five times, for different "feeling words" from the list. By creating a circumstance for a particular feeling, and creating a descriptive statement that characterizes your feeling, you will soon learn to listen for the feelings in words, even though the "feeling words" (like those in your lists) might never be spoken. Much of feeling expression is paralinguistic and nonverbal, and such practice will tune you into all of these dimensions of emotional expression.

After you have done five or more of these exercises, your interviewing partner should do the same, with you trying to identify your partner's feeling state at that moment from his statement. If you are wrong in your identification, your partner should correct you, which is quite like what might happen in an actual interview. With considerable practice, you should then move on to reflecting your partner's feelings, with words from the list, or that are not on the list, in actual brief interviews (2 to 3 minutes).

Following such practice exercises you should then deliberately engage in such counseling tactics in your regular 1-hour interviews with your long-term interviewing partner. This should then become a regular part of your repertoire of counseling tactics.

Summarizing Feelings

The process and tactics of "summarizing" a client's feelings can serve the same functions as "summarizing content." You can start off an interview by summarizing the feelings of an earlier interview. You may terminate an interview by summarizing the feelings expressed during a current interview. You may summarize a client's feelings after a segment of an interview to seek clarification, to determine if he wants to amplify any further, or to determine if he has completed his considerations and/or emotional expressions related to the circumstances that he had been talking about for the last few minutes. It should be remembered that reflecting a feeling focuses on the immediately preceding expressions, whereas a summarization of feelings involves providing the client with a succinct statement about his feelings that cover longer segments of the interview. As with summarizing content, you have to exercise some judgment about what might be the most significant feelings to reflect. You are not functioning as a tape recorder, but rather as a filter. If there is a pattern of feelings, or if certain feelings stand out above the others in terms of their significance, then you might limit your reflection only to those significant feelings. You are mirroring for the client what he has just revealed to you about his most intimate self. Your tone of voice and your language is critical in communicating your appreciation and sensitivity to the nature of what your client has just shared with you.

This process of mirroring your client's feelings serves not only to identify for the client any recurring patterns of feelings, but also the presence of any conflicts between feelings. Underlying all of this is also the function for the counselor that an accurate summarization of feelings can communicate to the client that the counselor "has been with the client" at his most private levels; that he understands even those things that are difficult to put into words. Such empathy shows the client that he is not alone in whatever his problem might be, and that he has available someone who understands, who can be trusted, but most of all, someone who will be and is a supportive companion in his search to understand himself and to change the way he communicates.

The process of summarizing feelings during an interview requires a quick, succinct selective function by the counselor. The client may have expressed a number of feelings, involving a number of diverse circumstances during a large segment of an interview. The summary by the counselor reflects, not each individual feeling, or circumstance, but rather some theme, pattern, or circumstance that binds the individual elements together in some meaningful way. For example, reflecting the diversity of feelings in a single circumstance can be a meaningful summary. Table B.1 in Appendix B provides a list of terms that may be helpful in labeling the numerous feelings we experience. It is provided in anticipation of difficulties that we may encounter as we try to put feelings into words.

Getting in touch with feelings is both a verbal and nonverbal process. The internal sensations, the external circumstances, and the verbal labels combine with one another as the total emotional experience. The client avails us of his words and body cues. He may also provide descriptions of external circumstances. However, the internal sensations, if true empathy is to prevail, must come from ourselves, from the counselor. For this reason, the counselor, as an accurate reflector of feelings, and to train himself in this process of reflection, might well get in touch with his own processes of emotional experience and expression. Getting in touch with our own feelings will develop an appreciation of the process, the resistances, and the experience that a client encounters during an interview, as he expresses emotional material.

However, there are additional functions to the recognition and expressions of the counselor's feelings. One of these can be accomplished through the tactic of "sharing" behavior, which is discussed later. Of relevance now is the role of the counselor's feelings in understanding his client.

From time to time during an interview, in addition to our reasoning and thinking, we may become aware of our own feelings. If we become aware of such feelings in ourselves, we should note them, and later outside of the interview, we should privately ask ourselves "What am I feeling about this person and about what he is presenting to me?"

Following this recognition, during this conference with ourself, we should then ask ourselves "Why am I feeling this way?" "What is the client doing to generate these feelings in me?" "What do I want to do as a result of how I feel?" "What does the client want me to do now that he has generated these feelings in me?" In this manner of getting in touch with our own feelings and self-questioning, we may develop an understanding of our client's feelings, motivations, and behaviors, as well as how our own feelings may be influencing the proceedings, that we might not otherwise perceive. A few examples may help:

1. "Why was I angry at the client? What is he trying to get me to do on the basis of my anger?"
2. "I feel sorry for him. Why? What did he say or do to make me feel this way?"
3. "What does he want me to do? Why does he want me to feel and behave in these ways?"

Finally, the process of summarizing feelings may have a very special defusing or safety valve function. It appears that an emotional experience can have several forms or perhaps phases. They may range from physical sensations and physiological activity, such as "chills," "the welling up of tears," and increased heart rate, to screaming and laughing and crying. When we attach *words* to these experiences in our primitive attempts to characterize them, like saying "I feel so good about this," or "I'm scared, really scared," it becomes a different experience. It now is translated from raw sensations to "cognitive coping." Putting a verbal label on an experience may be a first step toward managing it or understanding it. This idea of defusing an overwhelming emotional experience by labeling it has special applications if such experiences occur toward the end of a particular interview. Sullivan (1970) pointed out that clients should generally terminate an interview on a hopeful note and with feelings of self-worth and dignity. If an interview has been particularly heavy and the client, toward the end, is feeling down, unworthy, and anxious, the summarization of feelings by the counselor could help to reverse this state of affairs by the mere act of verbally labeling those feelings, either by him, or by helping the client to do so. Labeling is generally a cognitive process, and as such it represents, in some instances, a healthy tug away from overwhelming emotions. It is the two in combination (feelings and cognition) that may make for the most therapeutic experience.

Our job is to decide whether it is helpful for the client to understand what he is doing, how he feels about what he is doing, and how his various behaviors have been and will be influenced by such understanding. We can paraphrase the content or circumstances for the client's behavior and we can reflect his feelings back to him. We can also summarize his content and feelings.

Areas of content and feelings that have consistently come up during therapy interviews have dealt with the following:

1. The quick and easy change and control of speech—what it means, its durability, its implications for beliefs of victimization and helplessness, its short- term and long-term effects; the client's feelings about such change,

its meaning relative to labeling himself as having a speech defect, and relative to developing speech that is free of problems; and the development of deliberate monitoring skills.

2. Commitment to a schedule of therapy. The current distress of the client; problems of priority and motivation to change; new expectations and fears associated with problem-free speech; long-standing emotional investments in the problem.

3. Developing self-monitoring skills of the new speech behavior—resistance to becoming responsible for himself; overdependence on the monitoring of the clinician; the dualistic existence of error-free speech in the office versus errors outside of the office; general implications of self-responsibility in areas other than speech.

4. Environmental transfer of new talking skills—conflict and resistance; fear about error-free speech in the client's nonclinical environment; gambling on old behavior to see him through; tracking error behaviors instead of new behaviors; binding monitoring and deliberateness to expectancy of errors.

5. Replacing monitored speech with unmonitored, error-free speech—fears of reducing monitoring; juggling the schedule of replacement; maintaining motivation; changes in self-perception as a speaker; changing social roles.

Each phase of therapy, and those circumstances associated with therapy, constitute recurring experiences for the client. They can be areas of concern for the client. The client has different kinds of reactions and feelings to these experiences, and we have mentioned a few that seem to consistently need attention. We may well anticipate their occurrence. Our job as clinical interviewers and counselors is to reinforce the client's comments about these issues, to paraphrase his comments, and to reflect his feelings about these experiences so that he can clarify what he is doing and why.

When we are dealing with a focus on content, or on the circumstances for feelings, we paraphrase. This means putting the client's comment about the content into our own words, sometimes shortening it, or summarizing only the key elements of the content. It takes practice to do this easily and smoothly.

When we are reflecting the client's feelings, the source of information is everything the client might be doing at a given moment in therapy. It might not be what he says, but rather how he says it, loudly or softly, rapidly or slowly, or with a tremor in his voice. His body language, eye contact, and posture can all be a part of the emotional message; whether he's smiling or grimacing or crying. Feelings are often read from what is not said, but their reflection back to the client requires that the clinician develop a meaningful verbal vocabulary for characterizing these feelings. Again, it takes practice and experience, not merely reading about it.

We must help the client to keep his goals about changing his speech and his self-perception as a speaker (as a former speech defective if that is the case) in the forefront. Sometimes, a client's progress can be slow, sometimes it can be very rapid. Each of these circumstances can have the effect of reducing the client's motivation for pursuing the final phase of therapy, to gradually make his new skills automatic, so that they do not require any monitoring from him. He can become too satisfied too soon, and, as a result, never change his perceptions of himself as a special kind of speaker. Therefore, some of our tactics may be designed to ensure that the client fulfills his potential for progress. By reflecting the client's feelings we can communicate that we understand, that he is not alone, that we are supportive, and that we will help him through whatever obstacles there may be to reaching his goals, as long as he wishes to pursue them.

SUGGESTED PRACTICE PROJECTS

With your classmate or short-term interviewing partner, you might practice each of the functions that have been mentioned for "summarizing feelings."

Start off a mock interview with your classmate with a brief, succinct summarization of feelings associated with your previous interview with him. Of necessity, interviews for practicing "summarization" will be longer than your previous practice projects. Your partner will have to provide you with more material that lends itself to "summarization."

When the opportunity presents itself, insert a "summarization of feelings" that covers a segment of the interview (perhaps 5 to 10 minutes) to determine if all of the ground has been covered on that particular area of consideration; to ask for clarification; for amplification; and then finally as a way to terminate the interview. You might also practice combining such summarizations of feelings with summarizations of content; as a way of explaining patterns of feelings, their interactive dynamics, their consequences and effects on behavior, and the conflicts between feelings.

Following this type of practice with your classmate you should deliberately insert these "summarizations of feelings" tactics into your interviews, when they seem to be appropriate, with your long-term interviewing partner.

8

MORE ADVANCED INTERVIEWING AND COUNSELING SKILLS

Although the four interviewing and counseling tactics of *sharing, confrontation, interpretation,* and *clarification* are quite different from one another in a number of important ways, they are being grouped together here for preliminary discussion because of several overriding similarities.

Each of these tactics gets very close to those things that we do in our normal, everyday conversations with friends. However, their timely use in a clinical interview requires a very close monitoring that is quite different from their more spontaneous use in everyday interpersonal conversations.

Also, there is a movement in the focus of the material, be it emotional or cognitive, from the client to the counselor. The counselor's history, perceptions, theoretical and personal frames of reference, and personal needs in the relationship are introduced into the interview when these tactics are employed. However, there is a clinical "intentionality" that still relates to focus on the client, even though the material introduced may be tapping into material that relates to the counselor. As a result, they should be engaged in with caution, awareness, forethought, and deliberation. They may never and perhaps should not reach that automatic level of emission by the counselor that reflecting, paraphrasing, invitations to talk, and minimal encouragers do. Their appropriateness as facilitators for the client to understand and to change should be thought about, even though briefly, during an actual interview, before they are employed. It is this dimension of deliberateness and forethought that groups these four tactics together, although each one requires separate discussion.

SHARING

Sharing behavior refers to a tactic whereby the clinician shares something of himself, out of his own experiences of circumstances or feelings that he thinks will facilitate the process for the client.

The functions of sharing your own feelings, thoughts, and judgments during an interview are at least threefold. One function is to demonstrate your willingness to reveal to your client personal and significant material if it will be of help to the client to know these things about you. It shows that you are willing to do what the client does in this sharing experience, that is, to take a risk and to trust the confidentiality of the client, even though the ultimate focus is on the client.

Second, such personal sharing can demonstrate, with your own example, that you, the counselor, understand the nature and depth of the client's material by being able to translate it into your own experience. You really do know what the client is talking about and is experiencing.

Third, you give the client the message that he has a companion in the counselor, who by virtue of a similar experience has traveled the same road. Such companionship should minimize feelings of isolation, feelings of uniqueness, feelings that he is alone, or that he alone has known such problems. Although sharing behavior by the counselor focuses on material about himself, its ultimate function and focus is defined by the material brought out by the client, and is designed to help the client share material that may be difficult and painful.

The sharing that is employed by the counselor may be to show the client that he has had a similar feeling, or has been in a similar circumstance. But it is not a sharing of how the counselor resolved his problem. Sharing the resolution would not facilitate the independence and growth of the client.

Also, it is not the "gossiping" type of sharing that most of us engage in during our everyday personal conversations, when we unconsciously play the game of "Can you top this?"

Sharing behavior may come easily to some of us, perhaps too easily. It is not designed to relieve the tensions or meet the problem needs of the counselor. Sharing should be relatively brief and should not involve a long and detailed history or description about an incident. It should be long enough to accomplish its designated function, which is to facilitate the processes of the client. It should not result in a prolonged or specific focus on the counselor by either the counselor or the client. Most of us have probably shared the broad spectrum of feelings and emotions that characterize the human condition. Therefore, we have the common ground of experience available for emotional sharing. We each have probably experienced a sense of loss, moments of anger and frustration, as well as joy and relief and happiness and loving and being loved. We may not have experienced the same circumstances for these feelings, but this dissimilarity does not preclude the sharing that is possible about emotional material. For example, a sense of loss is the same or similar whether the circumstances for that feeling are associated with the death of a relative, a divorce, a child who runs away from home, or the end of an era, and so on. The client may report a sense of loss about one of these circumstances, whereas the counselor may share the same feeling about a different circumstance. In some instances all is common to both participants, and the sharing is that much more apparent and obvious to both. A very real sense of closeness can emerge from such sharing experiences during an interview and they can easily have a powerful empathic and emotional effect on both participants. It is not unusual for both parties to well up with tears as a part of the sharing.

An example or two might be helpful:

1. The client has just finished talking about how difficult it has been for her to accept the death of her mother. Her last statement was "I still can't handle it. I just miss her, not talking to her."
   Counselor (sharing): "I understand. I went through the same thing with my father. I sometimes feel that he is still with me, watching me, and even smiling."
2. Client: "I'm really so glad that my daughter lives so close by. But my son. I hardly hear from him anymore, he's 2,000 miles away, but not even a phone call." (she starts crying)
   Counselor (sharing): "I know what you mean. Both of my kids live out of town. It's not the way it used to be. It's hard to realize they're really on their own. But maybe there's a way to work it out and make it better than it is."

SUGGESTED PRACTICE PROJECTS

The practice projects for "sharing" can be divided into three stages. In Stage One, the goal is to get comfortable with the experience and process of sharing. In Stage Two, the goal is to get experience in "matching" your sharing to the material of your client. These two stages are done in a dissected fashion, outside of the interview situation. Stage Three is designed to provide experience in "matched sharing" during an interview.

The first practice project for learning how and when to share something from your own experience that matches the feelings and/or circumstances of what your client has or is trying to talk to you about, is to get comfortable with the process of sharing.

Either in a classroom situation, or alone with your short-term interviewing partner, your classmates and partner can be encouraged to volunteer to describe a specific emotional experience, providing both the circumstances and their feeling experience. These can range through all types of situations and feelings, positive and negative,

If it is done between you and your short-term interviewing partner, outside of a class, you should explain the nature of what you wish to practice. You can ask your partner to volunteer after you take the first turn. You should do this several times, sharing different kinds of experiences and feelings with each other, until both of you become comfortable with the process. At this point, you are not necessarily trying to match the other person's sharing, but rather trying to get comfortable with any type or manner of sharing.

In addition, after each instance of sharing and discussion, you should make an effort to "cut it in half." No matter what the length of your partner's or your own sharing was, yours should be succinct and to the point. After you have reduced the length of your own sharing several times, it should become easier for you to provide a brief sharing experience without the need to practice the shortening portion of it. You can then give up that part of the practicing.

Following this dissected exercise, with your classmate or short-term interviewing partner, you should continue with the mutual sharing between the two of you, but with the specific goal of "matching" the material presented by your partner. The focus for matching should be on the circumstance, the nature and depth of feelings, and the significance of the event.

In the Stage Three practice, you are to conduct an interview engaging in all of the tactics and behaviors that you have been practicing. When it is appropriate, try to insert a brief but on-target sharing experience of your own. It should not dominate the interview and become the subject for any prolonged discussion. The idea is to share so that it helps your interviewee over some rough material that he may have difficulty talking about, or to communicate that he is not alone or unique with his problem. Your sharing should not trivialize your partner's experience. Your sharing should demonstrate that you understand the depth and nature of what the client has been experiencing. It might be best to limit your sharing to one instance during the interview so that the focus does not shift from the client to the counselor, for either of the participants. Following these practice projects, you might then look for opportunities to engage in such sharing tactics with your long-term interviewing partner.

CONFRONTATION

Confrontation is a tactic whereby the clinician says something that can be perceived as aversive to the client. The client is brought face-to-face with some aspects of what he has been talking about that is not necessarily new material to him, but that is juxtaposed or related in ways that are new. This dimension of "newness" brings the tactic very close to the tactic of "interpretation." The difference between the two is that a confrontation only makes use of material that has already been introduced by the client.

Confrontations by the counselor often come about when a client contradicts himself, shows faulty reasoning, or reveals unproductive beliefs about himself and others that may be affecting him in very pervasive ways, for example:

1. Counselor: "You are smiling as you tell me how much you are afraid to talk on the telephone."
2. Counselor: "You tell me that you scream at your child to get him to stop crying, and that even though it isn't effective, you continue to scream."
3. Counselor: "Earlier you said that you would give anything to stop stuttering, but now you tell me there are certain advantages in stuttering."
4. Counselor: "You told me you didn't get the job because of your speech, but now you tell me that you didn't even apply for the position."

There is no doubt that certain self-truths can be aversive and that contradictions in the reporting of facts and thoughts, when pointed out, can be painful. For this reason, the counselor must decide whether a confrontation at that moment will facilitate or impede the client's growth.

Sometimes, a confrontation can provoke a client into his strengths of coping, for example:

Counselor: "You're telling me that you're helpless and feel victimized, like there is nothing you can do."

Client: "I know that's how I sound and I hate it; it's not the way I usually am or the way I want to be."

Confrontation should be employed cautiously. It can generate a great deal of emotion by the client, and can tap into depths of material that have not been touched on before. In addition, it can test the strength and trust in the relationship between the client and the counselor. However, when confrontation is engaged in, there is also an opportunity for the client to see that the counselor will not be "used," and that the counselor's warm but tenacious honesty will prevail. Such perceptions by the client of the counselor can serve as a model for the development of the same type of self-honesty in the client. However, we should remember that we as counselors must earn the right and privilege to confront a client. This privilege comes from the trust that the client has developed over a period of time.

As the counselor becomes aware of these types of issues, he has to decide whether pointing out some inconsistency at that moment to the client will be helpful to him. Confrontation is a risk because it can jeopardize the relationship if it is really punitive. At times, it may be best to delay confrontations until the counselor feels that the relationship is positive enough and strong enough to tolerate such tactics. Some clinicians feel that the timing of tactics differentiates a successful clinician from an unsuccessful one. The successful clinician knows when to confront and when not to confront a client. There is an "art of gentle pain" that comes with experience, so that eventually we know when a confrontation in a trusting and caring relationship can be effective.

SUGGESTED PRACTICE PROJECTS

This tactic of confrontation, in particular, should be practiced before it is used in an actual interview. Deliberately introducing aversive material into an interview without alienating the interviewee requires a great deal of skill with the language as well as sensitivity and warmth. Confrontation is not a hostile interaction. It is supposed to communicate persistence and honesty by the counselor in order to be more helpful to the client. To be helpful, it should enable insight and preserve the dignity and self-respect of the client. Such a challenge demands intentionality and practice.

Keep in mind that the counselor's goals are to confront, but in a warm and friendly manner.

With your classmate or short-term interviewing partner, the interviewee should be programmed to provide inaccuracies or self-contradictory content to give the counselor the opportunities to engage in several such confrontations during the mock interview.

After each confrontation, you and your partner should discuss what went on and how to improve it in terms of its length and acceptability. Examine the language, the tone of voice, the warmth, how it was approached. Then try the same confrontation again to see if the discussion had any positive effect. Do this several times, until you feel comfortable in doing it, and are able to do it briefly and with "affection" and "warmth." You may wish to add some types of qualifiers in what you say, to make it easier for the interviewee to accept your confrontation and still sustain your relationship and perhaps even "like and respect" you for doing it.

Following this type of "out-of-interview" type of practice you should practice engaging in such confrontational behavior with your long-term interviewing partner in a 1-hour interview. However, in these instances the confrontations will take place during the interview and will not be discussed or practiced in any dissected manner. You will have to look for and be alert for opportunities to confront instead of the "programmed" approach used with your short-term interviewing partner whereby he deliberately provided you with opportunities. This will be a much more real and spontaneous experience for your long-term interviewing partner, although it will still be an intentional, deliberate action on your part, with some forethought as to whether it would be helpful to your partner to have this experience.

INTERPRETATION

Perhaps the most sophisticated interviewing and counseling tactic is that of clinical interpretation. This refers to the process whereby a clinician provides new information or new understandings to the client. Interpretations by the clinician, although valuable, are not nearly as valuable as when the interpretations and understandings are generated by the client himself, in part as a result of his overall experience with the clinician.

By this we mean that the client sees himself, his problems, his ways of coping, his interpersonal relationships, and the relationships between seemingly uncorrelated events, in new ways that are quite different from the ways he had been previously understanding these issues. As a result of these new understandings, he may also see or understand in a new way how he was functioning in his here-and-now life. The depth of these interpretations by the counselor in part is defined by the degree of newness of the client's understandings, and in part by their pervasive significance and consequences as to how the client functions. Very often, a counselor may raise questions, reflect feelings, summarize content, confront, share, or juxtapose certain of the client's material content in an effort to help the client interpret himself to himself. The counselor tries to ease the client into these new self-perceptions and understandings. A self-generated and self-imposed insight may have a far greater probability of accuracy, acceptability, understandability, and durability. It also has the vulnerability of being filtered through the client's mechanisms of resistance and protecting himself. As such, these self-discoveries provide opportunities for the client to see himself in action during the interview. These defenses then also become available for scrutiny and further interpretation by the counselor and by the client.

The implication of this attempt to encourage client self-discovery is a strong suggestion that the counselor does not necessarily have to share immediately some new insight or understanding that he may have developed, but rather should give the client an opportunity to develop the same insight as a part of his growth.

The basic rationale for making interpretations to a client is that we, the counselors, have a point of view about the nature and dynamics of the client's problems; that we have some goals and objectives in mind for the client, probably both behavioral and conceptual (i.e., we have in mind that the client should feel, think, and believe certain things about the issues that are significant to him); that he should act in certain ways on the basis of these beliefs; and finally, that our own behavior of interpreting during an interview will facilitate all of these processes for the client. In other words, we know something that we think the client should know.

The issues considered in an interpretation offered by the counselor depend to a great extent on the training and theoretical perspectives of the counselor, and how he applies them to the material presented by the client. Several different clinicians could probably respond quite differently to the same material presented by the client, with each interpretation having its own validity within a particular theoretical framework.

As clinical interviews progress, the counselor may become aware of a pattern of thinking, believing, feeling, and behaving by the client. As he observes these recurring patterns of content, he may develop some hypotheses about their significance and what they might mean. It is much like employing the scientific method in a clinical circumstance. You observe something, you develop some questions and a hypothesis about what you have observed, then you go about making more observations, through your various interviewing skills, until you either reject or accept your hypothesis. This can lead you to a conclusion that you may decide to share with your client, which becomes your tactic or interpretation.

For example, your client tells you, "I quit school in my senior year because of my speech." On another occasion he tells you, "I didn't work for a long time, and just lived at home with my parents because my speech was so terrible." Then on yet another occasion he tells you, "I only hang out with guys, I don't know how to act with girls, because of the way I talk." At that point, you develop a hypothesis that your client is using his speech problem as a way of justifying many of the failing experiences he has endured socially, educationally, and occupationally. Then you go about questioning, inviting, and encouraging your client to focus on talking about these areas to see if the same pattern of explanation prevails. This type of scenario is rather common for people who stutter, and in this instance let us suppose that your hypothesis is verified. You now must face the real problem. Do you say to him, "You have been using your stuttering to explain away all of your failures," or do you keep on probing until he may say, "God, I've really made a mess of it. I'm blaming everything on my speech."

In the first instance, the counselor made the interpretation. In the second instance, the client is approaching the point where he is becoming capable of making a self-discovery, an interpretation of himself to himself, probably with further probing and encouragement from you, that he had other choices available to him while he was living with his communication problem.

In some instances an interpretation may relate the remote past to the present (e.g., "All of these years you have appeared helpless to yourself and to others because you were continuously told, or you told yourself, that you couldn't help the way you talked.").

At times an interpretation may correlate two or more events that had been perceived as quite discrete or unrelated (e.g., "You have selected your education, your occupation, your hobbies of working with your hands, with tools, with machinery, because you could be alone, and didn't have to talk to people, because you stuttered.").

At other times an interpretation may relate latent meanings of manifest material (e.g., "It sounds like what you're really saying isn't that you like being alone, but rather that you're afraid to reach out to people.").

Some of the content areas where clients have benefited from interpretations from the counselor, and that seem to come up quite often, include:

1. Exploring the client's need to identify the cause of his problem:

Counselor: There are many possibilities. What do you, deep down inside, think caused this problem with your wife?"

Client: "At first I thought she was embarrassed by the way I talked. But I don't talk like that anymore."

Counselor: "Maybe it has more to do with your improvement; that is, you don't need her to talk for you the way you used to. Maybe she feels generally that you don't need her or love her anymore."

a. Clarifying the sense of control he is gaining over himself:

   Counselor: "John, do you realize what you just did? You just made a phone call complaining about your newspaper deliveries, and explained it all with no errors of any kind in your speech."

b. Generally interpreting the course of therapy:

   Counselor: "This part of your therapy was easy. Now that you can speak the way you want to in here with me, you have to expand your operations, take your new skills to the outside world, to your family, at work. We've got to plan it out, the where and when."

2. Correlating the past to the present.

Counselor: "I know it's hard. You've been avoiding talking situations since you were a kid. Now you've got to face what you want to make out of your life. You've got the skills. The need or comfort to stay quiet and not talk is behind you."

3. Finding symbolic and latent meanings of what he is talking about:

Counselor: "I know that you're tired, and I know that you're afraid that you can't do it. You're not alone in this. Are you saying that you want to put your son in an institution, or that you want to work out a way to keep him at home with you?"

4. Correlating different current issues in his life:

Counselor: "You're really feeling down on yourself. A lot of bad things have been happening for you, and it's easy to ignore the good things that are happening. You lost your job. But you still have a loving girlfriend, a supportive family, and an outstanding education and work experience. Let's try to take it apart and put it together again."

5. Recognizing self-deception and less-than-honest thinking about himself and others (Shipley, 1992):

Counselor: "Maybe some of what you're feeling about yourself has to do with how long you've been living at home with your parents. You have a good job, so it isn't the money. You've blamed where you live for your lack of socializing with women. Honestly, John, I've known you for a long time now. I think it's an excuse. I think you've got a built-in excuse for avoiding that kind of socializing. There's something there that you're afraid to reach out for."

6. Accepting the fact that he has a problem:

Client: (follow-up to previous example) " You think I'm afraid of women?"

Counselor: "How many women have you spent any time with? From what you've told me, almost none. And yet you've told me that you've seen and met many women that you thought you'd like to be with. What's going on? Let's talk about this."

7. Recognizing the self-destructive nature of some of his own thinking, reasoning, beliefs, feelings, and actions:

Client: "I know that I get in my own way. I hear about jobs out of town and I don't go after them. I'm unemployed. I need a job, but I feel that I have to live here, and I don't know why. I don't have any friends here, just my parents, and I'm afraid to let go."

8. Recognizing the positive and facilitative aspects of some of the things he is learning in therapy (e.g., new speaking behaviors, new attitudes about speaking and social interactions, beliefs about himself and about others):

Counselor: "It sounds like you feel as though your therapy has been a good experience, even though there are still some loose ends."

Client: "Look, I know that I'm probably on borrowed time. But I can talk, I don't have any pain, and I'm living with my wife at home, on a good disability plan. We have enough to live on. You've helped me realize that my past life is behind me. But even though I can't handle that physically anymore, I've got a lot going for me, especially that group you got me into. It's one day at a time, but so far it's been good, and I'm learning to smell the roses."

9. Recognizing and accepting his strengths and his weaknesses (Haan 1977):

Counselor: (follow-up to previous example) "I'm in awe of your strength. You don't need your wheelchair anymore. Your speech is just about the way it was before your stroke. And I know that you're volunteering for different things in your community. Joe, you're amazing, and we could all learn from you."

In the process of your clinical and counseling relationship your client will reveal certain patterns of thinking, feeling, and behaving. With experience, these patterns become easily recognizable, because they are especially pertinent to living with a communication problem, or going through therapy for a communication problem.

The interpretive process means that you have introduced some material into the interview that is new, and that such material is designed to provide the client with new understandings, new self-perceptions, new ways of assessing and evaluating himself. Matarazzo (1971) pointed out that interpretations usually involve longer verbal outputs by the counselor and usually result in shorter verbal responses by the client. Perhaps the client needs the private time to assimilate, understand, and react both cognitively and emotionally to the counselor's interpretive comments before responding. As counselors we should learn to expect an interval of silence or a latency period before the client organizes an overt verbal response to an interpretation. We should also become alert to the nonverbal, emotional cues that may emerge, even as the interpretation is going on. Such things as tears, perspiration, smiling, change in gaze patterns, fidgeting, and so on, may tell us about the effects of our interpretation even before a verbal reaction is forthcoming. Interpretations can easily generate defensiveness, submissiveness, affirmation, anger, hostility, anxiety, or relief. They may escalate both cognitive and emotional responses that are on the verge of expression by the client.

Interpretation is typically engaged in more often by the more experienced clinician and counselor. It is reasonable and understandable that professional novices tend to avoid interpreting (though, unfortunately, amateurs do not) because of the large number of assumptions that underlie its effective use. Like sharing and confrontation, it is a deliberate counseling tactic requiring much forethought about its appropriateness and facilitativeness. It requires a confidence in the direction that the client is to move as a result of its use and that confidence may only develop in counselors after considerable professional experience.

At the same time, we should retain a welcoming and open mind to the interpretations offered by the client. The client's interpretations may cause us to revise our own understanding in very profound ways relative to the dynamics, tactics, and end goals for the client. It seems that interpretation can be a mutual process between participants that could result in a series of new understandings by both the client and counselor. They may combine and pool their resources and efforts in a truly dyadic union of thought, feeling, values, and reasoning. Such a mutual endeavor seems to be an outgrowth of the mutual respect, truthfulness, and trust that is the keystone of their relationship.

SUGGESTED PRACTICE PROJECTS

The forethought and intentionality of interpretation as well as the stages for developing an interpretation requires that you have tape recorded and analyzed previous interviews. These tape recordings of previous interviews contain the raw data from which an interpretation evolves. These data are the patterns of material presented to you over a series of interviews that have led you to ask certain questions about that material and to speculate about what they might mean.

There are several different types of practice projects that could be appropriate for the tactic of "interpretation" because they can mirror in a practice exercise the different aspects or phases of activity that are a part of this counseling behavior.

1. The first step is to observe closely what the interviewee is saying to the point that you are asking questions of yourself about what you have been hearing, and about how you are understanding what is being said to you. This can be done during the interview, by jotting down whatever

questions occur to you at the time; or immediately after the interview while you are listening to the tape recording and analyzing what is going on during the interview. These questions may relate to the various content areas and emotional states, suggested as frequently occurring in the previous discussion of interviewing. These questions should lead to a formal hypothesis on your part.

Initially, practice exercises in developing hypotheses arising from questions that are generated by what the interviewee has told you should be engaged in. This can be done by reviewing the tape recording of your previous interview with that partner. Hypotheses may deal with the relationships between events, rationalizing, patterns of emotional expressions, or seeing the functions of specific emotional reactions. The idea is to get yourself into a mode of thinking whereby your observation of the client leads to questions about how you understand those observations, which in turn leads to a hypothesis about some dynamic aspect that characterizes your client.

2. Following the practice in hypothesizing, you might now follow that up with practicing the techniques for "probing your client to gather evidence that either accepts or rejects the hypothesis." This means staying on a particular subject through minimal encouragers, questions, reflecting feelings, summarizing content, and the summarizing of both feelings and content, as long as you remain persistent in sticking with the same topic, until you are satisfied about the hypothesis you were verbally testing.

3. If the evidence provided through verbally probing your client supports the hypothesis, then you should practice the decision making that is involved in whether your client will benefit from acquiring this new information about himself. The actual practice activity is one of asking yourself what the consequences might be if he recognized or learned these new things about himself. Is it a part of his past that is no longer a part of the way he is now? Will it be painful for him? Will it help him in some ways? If the answer is a negative one, then it might be best to just drop that piece of information from what you are dealing with in the interview. You don't necessarily have to share each new insight you develop about your client, or force your client to see certain things about himself that might have a negative effect on him.

On the other hand, if the answer about the helpfulness of acquiring that information is "yes," then you need to decide whether you want to encourage the client to go through a self-discovery process whereby you help the client to learn what you have learned, but without coming out and directly telling him about it. You might think about how you yourself proved your hypothesis, and take your client through the same steps of observation, either through a summarization process alone or by redoing the open invitations and questions following your summarizations. A self-discovery experience, or in this instance a self-interpretation, can often prove much more acceptable, effective, and long lasting than an interpretation offered by you.

4. However, even with such practicing exercises you should still practice your own offering of an interpretation. The language should be simple and not full of professional jargon. It should be conducted with sensitivity to the fact that you are climbing inside this person, dissecting some parts of him, and sharing some very new perceptions about him. He will need your support, and warmth and concern for his well-being. He may well need time to assimilate what you have just told him, and may need some clarifying discussion, supported by the evidence you gathered during the interviews. This should not be a confrontation, but might well lead into a discussion of how helpful this information could be if he is to reach his goals,

He should not be put in a position of defensiveness, even if you both realize that he has been behaving in self-destructive ways, or he is ambivalent about accepting what you told him. He needs to be listened to, heard out, perhaps enabled to argue with himself, with your support throughout for whatever route he needs to travel in dealing with your interpretation. The trust you have developed with him is a prime factor in how this proceeds. He may even have some new information to offer to you that may modify what you told him. Both parties have to respect and trust each other during these very significant and intimate interactions. This type of counseling behavior is at the heart of Schweitzer's comments about our "intrusion into the modesty of the soul."

CLARIFICATION

Clarifications by the counselor to the client can come in many forms, either as separate declarative comments or explanations, or as part of other comments and responses that the counselor provides. Paraphrasing, summarizing, reflecting feelings, interpreting, and confronting—each can carry with it some clarification of ideas for the client. In those instances, where an explanation is embedded within these aforementioned tactics there is a dual function, of selectively focusing the client on some particular content or feeling, as well as explaining an issue to the client in a way that he had not conceptualized or thought of before.

Clarifying in this context refers to a process whereby the counselor explains the nature of an issue, which may extend the client's current or past understanding of that issue. It can sometimes be contained in the counselor's putting the client's comments into his own words, or it may be the result of the counselor explaining some totally new information to the client that he has previously misunderstood, in a declarative form. For purposes of learning and evaluating which particular tactic you have engaged in, we are suggesting that any declarative form of explanation that is not a part of some other counseling tactic be categorized as a "clarification." If it is combined with some other tactic, make note that you used that tactic as a way of clarifying (e.g., clarifying + paraphrasing). These occasions are listed in Table A.1 on the form for evaluating facilitative behaviors, in Appendix A.

A few examples of the various types of clarifying comments that could be made by the counselor are listed in Table 8.1.

Clarification, whether it is a simple declarative statement or is embedded in or is a part of another counseling behavior, is one of the most fre-

TABLE 8.1
Forms of Clarification

Declarative Clarification

Client: "I do not want my child to be singled out and taken for therapy from his classroom."

Counselor: "Mrs. Doe, I understand what you're saying. Let me explain how this happens. All of the children in the class are being screened to find out if they have a speech problem. If he passes the screening, that's the end of it. If it shows that he has a problem, we will get in touch with you to discuss what might be done. You will have to approve whatever actions may be recommended."

Clarification + Reflecting Feeling

Client: "I know you're trying to help, but taking my child out of class will make him self-conscious and not want the therapy."

Counselor: "I know you're concerned about him, but this is only a large group screening and he won't be singled out from the others."

Clarification + Paraphrasing

Client: "My son will not be taken out of his classroom for therapy. He'll be a laughing stock."

Counselor: "I understand. Of course you don't want him to be teased, but this is just a large group screening, No-one is singled out for anything."

Clarification + Summarization

Counselor: "I think I understand how you feel about this, Mrs. Doe, and I appreciate your calling and coming in to talk. If I understand what you told me, this is the first time you were ever aware that anything could be wrong with the way your son talks. Also, you were concerned that the school has been doing something with him that you wanted to be consulted about first.

"There's been a real communication breakdown here. The school routinely does a speech screening on all of the students. It doesn't mean that anything is wrong, we just want to be sure, and if we see anything that might warrant some special attention, we would get in touch with you to discuss it. That's really what this is all about."

(Continued)

TABLE 8.1
(Continued)

Clarification + Interpretation

Client: "I know there's something wrong with the way he talks. He gets quiet every time we say something to him about it. Ever since he started to talk he's been repeating words, and now for 2 years—he's almost 3—he's still doing it, but now he repeats sounds too."

Counselor: "You say he stops talking every time you remind him about it. And also his repeating words now includes repeating sounds as well. You know, a possibility, Mrs. Doe, is that his different ways of repeating might be related to your reminding him about it, or the way you remind him. Most children his age go through a stage of repeating words or sounds. It could be a part of his normal development in learning to talk and grasp the language. But maybe we ought to talk about a few other things that you might be able to do that could help this situation."

Clarification + Sharing

Client: "I don't know what to do. My 3-year-old boy is stuttering all over the place. My husband ignores it, but I just can't. I tried correcting him, but it seems to be getting worse."

Counselor: "I know just what you mean, Mrs. Doe. I just went through the same thing with my own son, and I'm a speech pathologist. None of us is immune, I guess. But then I remembered—even though I was worried about it—that most kids this age go through this as part of their normal development. It's a part of learning our language, and most of the time it just disappears. Maybe we can talk a little about how we can help to make that happen for you and your little boy."

Clarification + Confrontation

Client: "He does it all the time, at least every time I talk to him. He looks me right in the eye and repeats his words. He even smiles at me when he does it."

Counselor: "You say he does this repeating every time he talks to you. When do you talk to him? Tell me about your talking day with your 3-year-old.

Client: " When he wakes up, he comes into our bedroom and says 'Mama, Mama, uppy, uppy.' Then, as I'm changing him, and feeding him, he gabs away."

Counselor: "Think back, Mrs. Doe, to this morning—did he repeat words as he talked to you then, the way you said, or was he repeating to try to get your attention and to pick him up into your bed? And then while you were changing him, did he repeat again or not?"

Client: "Now that I think about it, he didn't."

Counselor: "So he doesn't really repeat all the time, does he?"

"One of the things that we should remember is that most kids go through this kind of talking as part of their normal development. It's part of learning to talk, and with most kids, as they develop those language skills, the repeating goes away. Let's talk a little about what his typical day is like, and what your day is like too. Maybe we can help this process along a little.

"What do you two do after you've dressed and fed him? Does he play on his own? Do you play with him or read to him? How much fun time do the two of you have with each other? How about his Dad—where does he fit into the picture, I mean in terms of spending time with him?"

quently occurring counseling behaviors. It is a cognitive activity, a reasoned explanation of something that appears to be not well understood by the client, but could be of overall importance to helping the client if he did understand. The counselor should follow the client's lead in assessing the need for clarification. If the client has no way of arriving at a particular understanding, because he does not have the necessary information, and if such information (as in the foregoing examples regarding institutional procedures) would extend his knowledge base and thereby affect what he feels about the situation, then such clarification could be extremely helpful.

On the other hand, if the counselor feels that the client may be capable of extending his understanding without the clarification, he should try to help the client do so. The focus might still be on what the client is feeling with or without the clarification, or prior to and after a particular clarification.

Cognition is not a substitute for examining how a person feels, or to be used as a method for dealing with feelings. But dealing with them in combination with each other could become a powerful instrument for helping someone understand himself.

SUGGESTED PRACTICE PROJECTS

With a classmate or your short-term interviewing partner, you can practice the tactic of clarification both within a mock interview and outside the interview, in a type of dissected exercise. The idea is to gain some experience in explaining.

These explanations could involve any number of themes. They might include something about yourself, or something you might have said during your interview with your partner, something about your interviewing partner, the nature of your interaction with him, about the dynamics of your respective roles and responsibilities during the practice interviews, about some aspect of the "rules of the game" (which can vary from circumstance to circumstance), regarding school, about the course you are taking, about the culture, or about some technical information that might be pertinent to the issues under discussion. These explanations should be offered in simple language, should not reflect any defensiveness on your part, and should not be done in any confrontational manner. Care must be taken that your explanation is not perceived as a judgment about the client, and that you do not appear to think he should have been able to understand without any help from you. The explanation should do what it is supposed to do—that is, to clarify something for the interviewee.

Outside of the interview, you might explain to your partner what you are practicing and share with him the various possibilities of themes that he might bring up that have some importance to him. Let him know that the focus for awhile is on clarification. Then give him a chance to raise some of these issues for you to explain. If you are unable to explain, don't fake it; merely let him know that you don't know, but maybe the two of you together can figure out a way to get at that specific theme or information.

Go through several of these explanations with him, and then reverse roles. But try to keep it all real, and deal with issues that have some significance for each of you.

Following this type of dissected practice, you might then get into a brief interview with your short-term partner, and if the opportunity for a clarification is presented, then engage in that tactic. It should be remembered that this is a tactic that is used if you think that the client will be helped if he acquires these new understandings. It does not have to be pursued if the information is not deemed to be significant or helpful.

9

SPECIAL EVENTS DURING THE INTERVIEW

At various times during interviews, certain events occur that seem to stand out from the others, and, as such, they deserve some discussion. They may or may not be special or different in their qualities, but they have a history of causing a certain amount of confusion or discomfort for counselors. For the most part, they seem to involve expressions of feelings and emotions, perhaps in ways that suggest that a person is being overwhelmed by his feelings, or is losing control of himself. The sensitive handling of such events by the counselor may be a key factor in the way the relationship between the client and the counselor develops and grows. Generally, the best thing to do at first when these things occur is just to let it happen. It's almost like handling a sailboat when you don't know what to do. Just let nature run its course, and see if it will right itself. Let go and let the person try to handle it on his own.

In all instances, as you have been analyzing each of the interviews with your long-term interviewing partner, you should be using the rear side of the evaluation form for writing descriptions of things that happened during the interviews that are not covered on the front side. You should be noting the themes that your partner has discussed, and anything unusual that might have occurred that you recognized or that impressed you. This is the place for writing down your impressions about yourself, your interviewee, and the relationship, as well as these special events. This will provide you with a quantitative as well as a qualitative analysis about your interviewing and counseling experiences with this person. It will also provide the basis for a pervasive analysis of changes that are taking place in you and your partner as a result of this counseling experience.

SILENCE

Most new counselors dread silence. They report that they feel stupid and confused during a silence, that they don't know what to do during a silence, that silences shouldn't occur, that they lose client focus and worry about their professional images, and that it is a reflection of their own incompetence.

Perhaps if we discuss the functions of silence by the client during the interview, some of these feelings, though understandable, will dissipate.

Some of the silence of the client may function much like the silence of the counselor. It may well be an invitation to the counselor to talk, to ask a question, and to take the responsibility or the lead for the verbal interaction. At other times, the client's silence could be a function of his organizing his thoughts and trying to put things into words. Sometimes he is trying to remember something he wants to tell you. Sometimes he is reacting privately to your comments. Sometimes he is thinking to himself, and his thoughts at this point in time are private and only for himself, and not for your ears and thinking and reactions. Sometimes it is an expression of hostility or a resistance to share himself with you. It is important to figure out what the functions of a particular silent interval may be, so that we as counselors can appropriately respond. It may merely be a pause, but if a silence lasts more than 5 seconds, the probability is relatively low of it being only a pause wherein the client will shortly continue to talk. If the client is pausing, you of course remain silent. If the client is organizing his thoughts, you give him every opportunity to put his thoughts into words by remaining silent. If his silence is an invitation to you to talk, you should not deny its function—you should comment or at least reflect that you understand what the client wants. If the silence suggests confusion, then you should revise your comment to make it more understandable. If the silence suggests a feeling (e.g., fear, resistance, difficulty talking about a topic, hostility, etc.), then you should help the client identify it and discuss it. Finally, if you do not understand the silence, then you should share your lack of understanding with the client.

SUGGESTED PRACTICE PROJECTS

In the chapter on Listening and Attending there was a brief discussion of "silent listening" as an important element in attending behaviors. However, these practice projects are somewhat different in that they take you several steps forward to gain some practice experience in "breaking the silence," and acting on what you think the functions might be of a particular silent interval by your interviewee. This type of practice can occur during the mock interviews with your short-term partner as well as with your long-term interviewing partner.

Several functions were mentioned previously in the discussion of prolonged silences by the interviewee. They included:

1. an invitation for the counselor to talk or take the lead
2. client is organizing his thoughts
3. client is trying to remember something he wants to tell you
4. client wants to keep his reactions private and not share them
5. client is confused
6. client is experiencing some type of emotional reaction (e.g., hostility, sadness, fear, shame, etc.) and is not ready to put the feeling into words.

It should be remembered that when you do nothing, you are still doing something. Remaining silent is an active process. It is an action on your client's part as well as on your part.

For numbers 2, 3, 4, and 6, the most appropriate thing that you might do is to remain silent yourself to give your client the opportunity to use his own silence without the interruption by your comments of his thoughts and feelings. However, after a prolonged silence you may wish to intervene with a comment that may either communicate what you think is going on for the client during his silence, or you might ask a question about what might be going on, or provide a reflection of what you think the client's feelings are during his silence, or communicate your own lack of understanding about the prolonged silence, with a minimal encourager such as "I'm not sure where we are right now."

However, if you are confident that the silence is a signal for you to take over, then you can take the lead, or comment that "You want me to take over now, don't you?" This can open up a discussion about his silence that could be very helpful in understanding its function.

CRYING

The most typical human response that most of us have to someone who is crying is to try gently to stop it, to make the person feel better about whatever he is crying about, to console, and somehow to communicate "that everything will be all right."

If we think about this, we of course become quickly aware that we are probably responding to our own discomfort as well as to the person who is crying, and also that we may well be engaging in "denial activity"; that is, denying that person's emotional expressions, his needs for such expression, or the validity of the circumstances that may be associated with these feelings.

It is quite possible that something hurts this person and that everything is not going to be all right. It is also possible that crying may be the first step in the direction of defining and accepting the reality of a situation. There may even be some emotional relief associated with crying, because the person may be finally acknowledging the hurt and all of the things that may be associated with it. For our own part, the best thing we can do is let the tears flow and support the person through his crying experience. Occasionally, we may find ourselves welling up with tears as we empathize with our client. Such reactions can only communicate our genuine concerns and understandings of the client's problems.

As far as the interview itself is concerned, we must show our respect for what the client is feeling in these instances, by acknowledging and reflecting the client's feelings, and once the tears begin to subside, to go on. Usually the client will comment on his own, sometimes with embarrassment and apologies, or by stating that he doesn't know why it occurred. If appropriate at that moment, we may help him acknowledge why it occurred. When the client shows that he is again gaining control, we can continue. However, we have seen many clients who continue to bring forth a great deal of meaningful verbal material right through their tears as they struggle to regain their composure. We may never get totally comfortable in the presence of someone who is crying, but we should learn to respect these times of emotions and to help the person understand their feelings and the circumstances when they occur.

It is not unusual for crying behavior to occur intermittently all through therapy sessions, and it is not always necessary to discuss or analyze it. There are times when it may be entirely appropriate to continue talking while accepting the tearfulness.

SUGGESTED PRACTICE PROJECTS

Crying is one of those spontaneous emotional experiences that you cannot easily program to occur. However it has been our experience that crying is a fairly common, spontaneous event during these practice projects because the participants are often sharing material that involves feelings of sadness, loss, and regret. When it occurs, it provides an opportunity for intentional practice of tactics that can be helpful to the person who is crying.

For practice purposes, can you increase the probability of crying? You probably can by introducing some content into your mock interview with your short-term interviewing partner. This is not recommended for actual interviewing, but as a practice tactic it can generate an opportunity for learning, and usually proves to be helpful to both participants.

You might suggest to your partner during one of your mock interviews to talk about loss. Let the partner set the specific circumstance for discussion, while you reflect the partner's feelings associated with that loss. If it results in a welling up, or tears, then you can engage in the appropriate supportive and encouraging tactics while not trying to impede or shut down this particular form of emotional expression. Do not be surprised if your own feelings match those of your partner.

If the circumstance doesn't carry the depth of feeling that generates crying, then you might suggest or ask if they ever experienced the loss of someone through death, and give them a chance to choose whether or not to discuss this with you.

Again, you should reverse roles with your partner so that you also have the emotional experience of working through such an experience while sustaining your intentional counseling tactics.

EMOTIONAL EXPRESSIONS TOWARD THE COUNSELOR

It is tempting to discuss this topic within the theoretical perspectives of "transference." From a psychodynamic standpoint, transference is what therapy is all about. By transference we are referring to that process whereby the counselor becomes the object for, the target of, and the symbol of the client's emotional expressions and emotional relationships, past and present. It is natural that as a therapeutic relationship develops more deeply (in terms of speech and/or counseling), we generate and gain the client's trust. As the client is guided through various stages of self-understanding and change in self-perceptions and behavior, and as partners not only in counseling but in changing the way the client talks, in this total experience, the client and the clinician will be relating to each other in significant and meaningful ways. It will in all probability cover the broad spectrum of feelings, both positive and negative, by both participants.

From the clinician's standpoint he shares only those of his own feelings that facilitate the client's therapy. Any other feelings that the counselor may have are kept private and not inserted into the interview.

However, most, if not all of the client's emotional expressions are free to occur and are usually encouraged to occur. We should expect the client's anger and hostility as well as his love and affection. We also have to understand the functions of these expressions and, when appropriate, to interpret their meanings to the client. Anger and hostility may come early or late, as well as love and affection. Their interpretations in terms of the person's problems and in terms of the processes of therapy can be very helpful, and sometimes necessary if therapy is to progress. Emotional expressions toward the clinician usually requires that the client feels comfortable enough to do so. Often in the beginning, as significant issues are first approached, we may see negative feelings of self-protection. Later, after a significant sharing, or after significant insights and changes have emerged, the expressions may be quite positive. As a client moves from his initial needs for nurturing and dependence to his later needs for independence, we may see comments that suggest a more mutual or peer relationship.

These expressions can take many forms, from simple personal questions about the counselor's family and home life, to romantic inclinations and seductiveness. In fact, these experiences may come quite early in the working relationship, while the roles of each are being experientially defined. When two people are partners in helping positive changes take place in the life of one of them, it is only natural that strong (nonromantic), healthy bonds of affection will develop between them.

We should look for and be alert to these expressions of feeling toward us, try to understand their functions, and become comfortable with their occurrences in therapy. They are not threats to our personal integrity, to our professional credentials, nor to our personal needs. We should not run away from them, we should not deny their genuineness, and our handling of them should both preserve the therapeutic relationship as well as the dignity of the client.

SUGGESTED PRACTICE PROJECTS

Practicing tactics for dealing with emotional reactions toward the counselor can move in many different directions, depending on whether these reactions are positive or negative. For the counselor, they should be understood within a framework of looking for latent meanings, and trying to understand what is motivating the client's expressions of these feelings.

Often, the bonds of affection that come out of this partnership involve gratitude, respect, and a certain kind of nonromantic love that comes from feeling close to someone that you trust and have revealed yourself to. The counselor has to be sure that such expressions are not a part of overdependence on the counselor, or a shifting of responsibility to the counselor, or a mistaken romantic fantasy. You need experience in dealing with such emotional expressions when and if they ever arise.

With your short-term practice partner look for such expressions during your interviews with him. If they do not occur, let him know that you need to get some experience with this type of material, and ask him to deliberately tell you about the things he likes about you. This will give you the experience you need in accepting or rejecting them, without defensiveness, or embarrassment, and with sensitivity toward your client's dignity and good feelings about you.

Following this, then ask your partner to tell you about some of the things he doesn't like about you, about what you do during the interviews, or about the experience he has been having with you. Again, you will have the experience of dealing with this material in a way that is helpful to your partner. The problem for you is to maintain your focus on the interviewee, no matter how personal he may get. This is a type of desensitization process, where you get bombarded with distracting material and still try to maintain your focus and engage in helpful yet sensitive counseling tactics.

CONCLUSION

Thus it is within this total context of the therapeutic relationship that the structure for therapeutic change is established. It is within this relationship of initial respect and honesty that the client has an opportunity to lay away the past, to talk about the meaning of change, to integrate his new speaking skills into a new self-perception as he experiences himself in society, seeing himself as a new and different speaker and perhaps as a person who is quite different from the person who first started therapy. This is the substratum that makes conditioning of speech more than a laboratory exercise or a game to be played, limited to the clinician's office. The relationship with the clinician, and the opportunity to look at the social and emotional meaningfulness of the changes in speech may be the difference between relapse and permanence of outcome. It is a therapeutic view of the possibilities for combining these concepts into a powerful and effective therapeutic experience.

It becomes apparent that the speech pathologist must wear several hats, almost simultaneously. As a teacher, he may be instructing or providing examples for his client about how to emit a particular motor speech response. As a reinforcer, he may be strengthening desirable and weakening undesirable elements of talking behavior. As a counselor, he may be helping his clients to develop an awareness of the significance and implications of his changes in talking behavior, hopefully to the point where the client has learned to like himself and be comfortable with himself. Thus, the speech pathologist may move in and out of these "instructor"/

"counselor"/"reinforcer" activities at his own discretion, from moment to moment, as the needs of the client seem to dictate. The tactics of counseling may be interrupted if it seems appropriate to focus for an instant on some aspect of the client's motor talking behavior. We may well have a number of apparent discontinuities as these vacillations between "counseling" and "instructing" and "reinforcing" occur and recur. However, even in these vacillations, the focus is always on the client; we are always working toward generating trust, generating a positive expectancy, and facilitating change and self-expression as well as self-understanding, self-discovery, and self-actualization by the client. Both the client and the clinician have to learn to become comfortable with these several roles and patterns of clinical activity by the clinician. The warm and trusting relationship and the experiences that build up between the client and the clinician should eventually enable both participants to move in and out of these elements of the relationship with relative ease and comfort.

We must give the client every opportunity to reason, understand, develop insight, and interpret for himself. This kind of growth is as important as his changes in speech, and we must be careful not to permit the client to become overly dependent on our thinking, but to see the value of depending on himself for honesty and self-evaluation, for self-exploration and appropriate action. We are trying to promote a certain amount of independence and problem-solving ability by the client, so that he can give up his helplessness and learn to manage his problems with less and less intervention by the clinician. We want him to reach that point where eventually he does not need us for anything. He will know the behaviors he wishes to maintain, be able to monitor his speaking, be able to evaluate his actions, and become generally responsible for himself to the point where he will not require special professional support for dealing with the stresses he may encounter in the future. It is within this context of mutual commitment, support, interpretation, and professional companionship—including the tenacity and honesty of the clinician—that the behavioral aspects of speech therapy take on their overall clinical effectiveness and social importance.

10

FACILITATIVE HOLISTIC ATTRIBUTES OF THE COUNSELING INTERVIEW

For purposes of discussion, the holistic, nonspecific aspects of counseling are divided into two parts and are considered separately from the specific facilitative behaviors. This chapter deals with holistic facilitative or desirable attitudes and behaviors. These are listed in Table A.2 in Appendix A, whereas chapter 11 and Table A.3 in Appendix A deal with nonfacilitative or undesirable holistic attitudes and behaviors. Both are considered nonspecific, or holistic, because our assessment of them is based more on subjective judgment of large segments of the interview, sometimes of the interview as a whole, rather than on objective counting of individual occurrences of behaviors.

Although we might be able to identify and count elements of specific behaviors that relate to them, the micro-elements of behavior are not the same as these more holistic factors.

The list of attributes in Table A.2 is not an exhaustive one. There may be a number of other categories that readers may wish to add that contribute to the effectiveness of the interview. These characteristics focus on the interviewer. But there also may be some value in your creating a list of factors that characterize the client such as "resistance," "transference," "is often overly emotional," "dependent," "nonexpressive," "flirtatious." These attributes of the client can also affect the nature and effectiveness of the interview, and could be considered in an ongoing evaluation or description of the relationship. It is suggested that such client holistic factors (positive and negative) should be noted, described, and written down on the reverse side of Tables A.1, A.2, and A.3, so that you can analyze and integrate their occurrence into your overall analysis of the series of counseling interviews.

The goal of this commentary is to sensitize the reader to the numerous nonspecific things that can and should be looked at if we are to understand the processes of interviewing and improve ourselves as interviewers.

Interviewing and counseling is dynamic and usually dyadic. It is an active process where both parties participate as listeners and talkers. At times, the clinician may be totally silent while nonverbally attending, as the client verbally responds to each of his own preceding utterances and thoughts. At other times, the client may be silent as the interviewer offers his facilitating comments. If we wish to recognize the effects that the participants have on one another during interviews and to determine their desirability, then a first step is to become aware of the existence of nonspecific attributes of the interview. These holistic attributes often evolve and become characteristic of the interview as a result of the more specific behaviors of the counselor. Some of these attributes characterize the individuals, some characterize the interaction, and some characterize the relationship. Furthermore, as we look at more specific interviewing tactics and behaviors, these nonspecific attributes may become valuable in assessing the desirability and effects of the specific behaviors, as they may relate to the nonspecific attributes. Perhaps the final validity of our specific interviewing behaviors lies in these relationships between nonspecific and specific interviewing behaviors.

In Table 10.1, the listing of these facilitative, holistic attributes also includes some examples (out of context) of how they may be expressed during an interview.

However, we need some operational definitions and an appreciation of the goals and functions of each of these holistic attributes if we are to recognize them.

Client Centeredness (Person Centeredness)

This refers in part to the counselor's focus on the client. But beyond that, it requires that the counselor arrange the conversation so that the client takes the lead, and sets the agenda, so that the client gets comfortable in taking risks of revelation, sees his own responsibilities in the counseling process—in other words, the counselor sets the stage for the client's self-discovery and self-actualization. It means that through his silence the counselor invites the client to take the lead. He also sets the stage for the client to take the lead through his open questions, through his open-ended instructions, and through his verbal and nonverbal encouragement to talk. It is an overall attitude by the counselor that is supported by his words and actions: that he values the client's version of his problems, and values what the client talks about and wants out of the counseling process.

SUGGESTED PRACTICE PROJECTS

A valuable practicing project for learning client centeredness can be arranged with a classmate or with your short-term practicing partner, whereby you again role play being the counselor as well as being the client. During this short (perhaps 10 minutes in length) interview, after an initial open invitation to the "client" to talk, you let him know that anything that he wants to talk about is appropriate, but that it should be about something of some importance to him. The counselor's role is to stay focused on what the client is talking about. All invitations or questions or requests for clarifications—all comments—should relate to the topic chosen by the partner. You may be silently attending, actively listening, providing encouragement to your partner to continue talking. Limit yourself to that type of behavior as much as possible, so that your partner is leading you, instead of you leading him.

Accepting

This relates to the previous attribute. It means that the counselor receives and welcomes the client's leads, and communicates that he understands what the client is talking about and is experiencing. It functions to communicate to the client that the counselor wants him to continue in taking the lead and setting the agenda, that the counselor trusts the client's judgment about what is pertinent, and is willing to continue in this mode of client leadership, responsibility, and self-discovery.

SUGGESTED PRACTICE PROJECTS

A valuable practice project for learning to be accepting is quite similar to the previous one. It involves adding to the mix some verbal and nonverbal indications that you understand what the partner is talking about. This can easily be accomplished by paraphrasing, or putting into your own words what your partner has just told you, or by reflecting the partner's feelings. Also, such encouragers as "I see" or "I understand," or nonverbal "head-nodding" communicates your understanding and acceptance of what was just said to you.

The roles of counselor and partner should again be reversed so that you get a feeling for what you are trying to get your partner to do.

Fluent

This refers to the counselor's style of responding, both verbally and nonverbally. It suggests a smooth flow of speech without any tentativeness or irregular pausing and interjecting. This attribute tends to foster confidence in the client that the counselor is in tune with the client.

SUGGESTED PRACTICE PROJECTS

A practice project for this attribute of demonstrating your fluency again involves a brief role-playing 10-minute interview, as well as switching roles. In this instance, one way of communicating your fluency (or lack of tentativeness) is to try to avoid asking any questions. It suggests a fluency of thought as well as a fluency of speech. Again, paraphrasing content and reflecting feeling, or clarifying an issue for the partner, can demonstrate that you know where you are and where you're going, relative to what your partner is talking about during the interview. In this instance, the partner might be programmed to pause after he has made a comment, to give the counselor an opportunity to practice demonstrating his fluency.

Concerned and Empathic

We hesitate to suggest any hierarchy among these holistic attributes, but this particular attribute is one basic building block for the entire process of counseling (as perhaps each of the others are as well). It refers to a process whereby the counselor identifies with the client, and tries to think and feel the way the client does; to walk around in his shoes and in his world for a few minutes. This may not be easy or pleasant for the counselor to do, especially if the counselor privately doesn't totally admire what the client is doing, thinking, or feeling.

SUGGESTED PRACTICE PROJECTS

A way of preparing yourself for learning how to become more empathic and concerned involves a process of imagining yourself in a particular type of situation. You might try to imagine yourself in the role of someone you admire—a celebrity, an athlete, an actor or actress, a singer or musician, a friend or professional person you know. Imagine that person in a specific situation. Go through the actual imaging of it—the person, his face and expressions, his voice, what he is doing. Shut everything else out and imagine him. See, hear, and feel that person in that circumstance.

What would you feel if under certain circumstances, you were that person—not in terms of problems, but in terms of that particular circumstance?

Try to imagine yourself in that partner's specific situation, being that person in action. In order to do this you have to close your eyes and shut everything else out. Focus your thoughts, your visions, and your hearing on that person's face and voice in that situation. For example, if your partner were a speech pathologist, imagine that after a particularly good therapy session, his client said to him, "I will never forget you, what you've helped me to do"; and then she kisses him on the cheek, and says "Thank you, I will never forget you."

After you have imaged your partner in that situation, then imagine yourself being in that role of the clinician. See the faces, hear the words, see the action. What do you feel? What do you think? What do you do? Describe it. Put it into your own words, out loud. If you are with your practice partner, tell him these things. If you are alone, say all of this into a tape recorder, and then listen to it.

After you've done that, then try to do the same thing for something positive that your long-term interviewing partner may have told you in a previous interview. Now do the same thing for something he told you that is negative, that you don't agree with. Imagine it in its entirety, the words, the circumstances, the feelings. It takes doing and it takes practice. You might play a tape recording of some portion of an interview that you've had with him. Listen to the words, to the tone, to the feelings, and repeat them to yourself. In a sense try them on for size, see how they fit you. Can you throw yourself into your client's shoes, feel what he felt at that moment? It takes time to do this (between interviews, of course), but it can help you to experience whatever feelings your client was experiencing and prepare you to empathize more easily during your next interview with him.

Sometimes role playing with another person (a classmate or friend, not with your long-term interviewing partner), where you switch roles, will bring it to life for you.

You can take the role of one of your parents, or your spouse or the significant other in your life, or your boss, under a particular circumstance. As you throw yourself into that circumstance as that person, you will begin to experience what that person might be feeling under those circumstances. Then you might role play being your client, and let another person be you in a brief role-play experience.

Once you are able to get into your client's role to the point that you really know and appreciate where he is, it is important that you communicate your understanding to him. If you can do this, he will learn to trust you even more, be even more open than he has been, and gain even more confidence in what you and he are doing together to help him resolve his problems.

There may be some occasions when the material is so repugnant that you aren't able to empathize because your own negative feelings take over. In these instances, a desensitization procedure might be helpful, wherein your partner literally bathes you in the negative content, as you try to maintain your helpful attitude and execute helpful behaviors even as you are experiencing this repugnant barrage from your partner.

Relaxed and Calm

There may be many occasions that call for the counselor to be relaxed and calm. The chief function of showing one's calm during an interview is to communicate to the client that no matter what level or type of excitement or emotion the client introduces into the interview, the counselor is capable of understanding and dealing with the situation in an effective manner. He does this by staying with his style of communicating. He makes sure that there are no sudden and abrupt changes in his tone of voice, in his fluency, in his rate of speech, or in the loudness level of his speech. The paralinguistic aspects of his speaking remain constant and steady.

Sometimes the client is overwhelmed by his feelings and emotions. On such occasions, the calm of the counselor should not be an attempt to lower the excitement level of the client, because that level of excitement may have some significance for both the client and the counselor. There may also be occasions when the client is directing his emotional remarks, either positive or negative, at the counselor. The counselor's relaxed demeanor during such emotionalism again communicates his acceptance and willingness to look at what the client is doing at that moment, and that he, the counselor, does not enjoy any special or privileged immunity from the client's remarks, and also that he has not been caught up in the client's remarks to the point of letting his personal reactions become inserted into the situation.

The counselor's calm and relaxed style is not meant to be a role model, so that the client adopts the counselor's calm during his sessions with the counselor. The counselor may well wish to comment about that if the client somehow communicates to the counselor that is what is happening. The counselor's relaxed, calm, style keeps things moving in a helpful direction, even in the face of the client's continued emotionalism and excitement.

SUGGESTED PRACTICE PROJECTS

Again, an appropriate practice project for remaining calm and relaxed would be a desensitization role-playing experience with a classmate for several minutes, wherein your classmate literally bombards you with extremes of emotional outbursts, some of which might be directed at you, while you deliberately maintain your calm poise, listening, maintaining focus, and engaging in appropriate interviewing behaviors (Wolpe, 1986).

This can be approached in a hierarchical manner, by starting out with relatively calm interactions, and gradually the interviewing partner increases the excitement level to almost distracting levels. As preparation for this type of desensitizing, you could provide your partner with a list of five or six events or topics, from unexciting to very exciting, and your partner could spend time on each of these, making it more and more difficult for you to maintain your calm. If you "lose your cool," then back the conversation down to a less-exciting level, recover your calm, and try to reapproach the more exciting material. When you and your partner have taken turns at this desensitizing process, each of you should engage in a 2-minute interview in which either of you is free to introduce such material into a mock interview situation. Following this, you should be able to handle such events if they come up during your interviews with your long-term interviewing partner.

Does Not Interfere or Impede

This refers to the counselor giving the client a continuing opportunity to present himself, with minimal influence of the counselor. Usually, the total amount of talking time (if that is measured) will reveal who is dominating the talking during the interview.

Interruptions, questions, requests for clarification, and topic changes by the counselor can interfere with the direction that the client wishes to pursue. Such actions by the counselor may be more effective after the client has completed what he has started without such impedance by the counselor. There will always be an opportunity to influence the client later, if he has moved into irrelevance or has wandered away from his original premises and issues.

Once a client gets moving in his risk taking and talkativeness, and starts meandering through his world—through some associative chain of thoughts and feelings that are not quickly apparent—you never know where the client may take you. Sometimes he leads into some unanticipated depths of considerations that he may not have otherwise wandered into. The counselor should permit such free associations and mental explorations without the hindrance of some perceived need for the client to go where he thinks the counselor wants him to go. Although the counselor has a responsibility for influencing the content of the interview, it is a shared responsibility with the client, where the client may and should have a larger share of their partnership. The counselor's behavior may well be limited to his silence, or nonverbal encouragement such as head nodding, or very brief verbal encouragement. Each of these usually communicates to the client that the counselor wants him to continue.

SUGGESTED PRACTICE PROJECTS

In those instances where the task is to recognize something that you do not want to do, the process of negative practice can be helpful. You learn to recognize what you don't want to do by actually deliberately doing it (Dunlap, 1932).

This particular holistic attribute of not interfering or impeding may be one of those occasions where negative practice would be appropriate.

As a practice project, with your short-term partner, deliberately engage in some of those behaviors that you think may impede or interfere with the client's interview. Observe what the effects are of changing the subject, interrupting, denying a feeling, or judging. Also try to get in touch with your own feelings as you do these things. Such an experience may enhance your sensitivity to those effects, and also enhance your ability to recognize immediately when you may have engaged in them in your interviews with your long-term partner.

Does Not Judge

This issue has a direct bearing on how much the client will eventually trust the counselor. To expect someone to entrust, without any editing, all of the things that they would never entrust to anyone else, carries an expectation that the client's feelings, past history, current thoughts and actions, things they might feel guilty or ashamed of, are not being put on trial for the counselor to pass judgment on, whether they are right or wrong or reasonable or unreasonable. The client's logic and feelings and morals are what they are. They may change, they may even need changing, but judging them is not the issue or the vehicle for accomplishing these goals. This is true even when the client may be asking the counselor to pass judgment on him. The counselor's function is to help the client understand himself in relation to these issues, to recognize where his ideas and beliefs and feelings may have come from, and to see their helpful or destructive dynamics and consequences. It is the client who will judge or not judge. It is the client who has to see or discover the need to change something. Sometimes, just telling someone about something you may feel guilty about, or ashamed of, or afraid of, can be a most significant helpful first step toward these goals. The counselor's judgments can easily jeopardize the entire process.

The trust that emerges, the closeness that evolves, as a result of one person not judging another person's disclosures and risk taking may be one of the most significant and powerful aspects of their interaction. It may well set the stage for looking at things together that might be quite painful, if the client knows that he will not have to face them alone, but rather with an understanding, compassionate companion.

Judging someone else can sometimes happen too automatically, too quickly, and sometimes very subtly. Sometimes, without thinking, a counselor may say something that can be perceived as a judgment. Often a client seeks approval from the counselor. This is a form of asking for a judgment from the counselor.

Being supportive is not the same as being judgmental. Being supportive is not the same as giving approval. Saying that you understand is not offering a judgment. Being supportive of someone's expression of feelings does not imply a judgment of the validity of those feelings.

SUGGESTED PRACTICE PROJECTS

Here again is an instance where a few minutes of negative practice might be helpful, during which you role play an interview with your short-term partner and deliberately provide positive and negative judgments about what is being told to you. You can also contrast them with being supportive.

Also, you should switch roles, so that you each experience the effects of being judged, or of having a judgment withheld where there has been a history of judgment and approval. Such negative practice should again sensitize you to when these instances may have occurred during your outside interviews with your long-term interviewing partner, and also provide you with an appreciation of what it feels like to be judged.

Does Not Give Answers or Suggestions

This particular holistic factor fits in with the goal of self-discovery and self-actualization. One of the many goals of counseling is to help a client discover for himself, from himself, not only the nature of his problems, but also the possible resolutions. If the client depends on the counselor to resolve, to give him answers, to tell him what to think, what to feel, and what to do, he may never take on that responsibility for himself, and may forever be in need of someone to do that for him. The counselor can lead the client to these self-discoveries in many ways, even calling on some of his own experiences, but only to the point of helping the client to take the next big steps on his own. The client may benefit from having the counselor share some of his own similar experiences, but only if it results in a feeling by the client that he is not alone or unique in the issues he is considering, and as a result that he is in the company of someone (the counselor) who has been there, and understands. But the client then has to apply what he has heard from the counselor to himself. What the counselor never shares is how he, the counselor, resolved these similar issues for himself. The client may well ask the counselor to tell him how he resolved these problems. This can be a rather seductive request, because it may unconsciously appeal to the counselor's ego needs to be the authoritative expert who knows how to fix everything. Or, the counselor may actually feel that "his way" would be the best for this client, even though he recognizes the possibility of other choices.

It is incumbent on the counselor to explain that his resolution may not be the only resolution available, and that his resolution may not be the one for the client. But more importantly he should explain that he, the client, must try to figure it out for himself if he is ever to become free and independent of outside help. The counselor should further explain that the client isn't facing the search for a resolution alone, but that he will still be there to help him sort it all out.

SUGGESTED PRACTICE PROJECTS

The practice projects for this attribute (giving answers and suggestions) can involve both positive and negative practice.

Again, with your short-term interviewing partner, and by switching roles, the "client" can be programmed to ask the counselor for suggestions and advice and answers, again and again during the short interviews. This gives the "counselor" the opportunity to decline and to say those things that will encourage self-discovery and self-responsibility in the client.

For the negative practice portion of the exercise, given the same programming for the client, and even without it, the counselor can deliberately give advice, suggestions, and answers, but the client, in turn, should be programmed to push for more details about the suggestion (e.g., "Then what do I do?"), forcing the counselor to see how he is enabling helplessness and dependence. He will also see how he is not only intruding on the client's growth, but is being dragged into a scenario that totally subverts his role and his purpose as a helper.

Does Not Deny Feelings

Another way of stating this holistic attribute is that the counselor accepts the feelings of the client. One way of doing this is for the counselor to state what he believes the feelings of the client were, if the circumstance was in the past, or are, as the client is expressing them in the here and now during the interview. By putting the client's feelings into words, the counselor shows that he understands what the client is experiencing or has experienced. The counselor certainly doesn't tell the client that he shouldn't feel that way, that he should feel some other way, that the feeling isn't appropriate, or that time will change it. That is not accepting the feelings of the client.

The counselor may reflect the client's feelings, thereby accepting them. He may put them into a context of a particular situation or circumstance in the hope that some kind of understanding of the feelings will emerge, and he may help the client to see how these feelings may be affecting the client and his relationships with people. People act and relate in our society on the basis of what they believe and feel. Living with a communication problem, or with any kind of problem, generates beliefs and feelings that influence what we do. The effects of feelings can have wide-sweeping and pervasive significance, including effects on our life goals, our education and occupation, our social functioning, as well as our own sense of self-worth.

Feelings are the poetry of the mind, the engine that makes us go and do, or stop and avoid. They can entangle us into never knowing or embrace us into learning all.

Our sense of being at peace with ourselves, of liking ourselves, or of self-disgust, our anger, even violent feelings—we can feel all of these, and each can drive us to act in certain ways and to relate in certain ways. Understanding these forces and relationships, and utilizing these understandings to make appropriate changes—to go from negative to positive in how we cope with the many nuances of our human condition—is really what counseling is about.

SUGGESTED PRACTICE PROJECTS

The practice project for this attribute of not denying feelings is one of learning to reflect feelings. Not all feelings are expressed explicitly in words by the client. Much of it is paralinguistic or nonverbal.

Again with your short-term interviewing partner, in a brief mock interview, after your opening invitation to talk, try to limit yourself to only reflecting feelings. Don't paraphrase, don't ask questions or do any more inviting, only reflect feelings. Focus and concentrate, for these few minutes, only on what your partner is feeling.

There is an additional and detailed practice project associated with reflecting feelings that is considered in chapter 6 on Specific Facilitative Interviewing and Counseling Behaviors that relates to this practice project.

Absence of Self-Focus

The absence of self-focus refers to the counselor's attitude and behavior. The counselor concentrates and centers on the client and the issues that are pertinent to the client's problems. Even though the counselor approaches such a focus with a keen awareness of himself and his role in the counseling process, he does not insert into the interview issues that focus on himself. The main function of such a focus is to communicate that the client is the most important object of attention during this period of time. It communicates the concern of the counselor, the valuing of the client by the counselor, and the self-subordination of the counselor. There are many things that the counselor can do to enhance these perceptions by the client. The most obvious is that the counselor does not tell the client about himself, or about similar circumstances he may have experienced that are much like the client's, unless it is a deliberate "sharing" tactic designed to help the client reveal various issues to the counselor. He should not get involved in "chitchat" about things that he has been doing or thinking that have little to do with anything going on during the interview. The counselor's life is his own, and should remain private and kept out of the client's sessions. It is not the subject of discussion, and is not the reason the participants are spending time together. Such absence of self-focus will also help the client see that he is the "subject," and through such subordination of the counselor, that the client has a responsibility to move into the role being developed for him.

SUGGESTED PRACTICE PROJECTS

Again, role playing with your short-term interviewing partner is the vehicle for practicing. In a brief interview of perhaps 10 minutes length, start off with some type of invitation to talk. It might be a time to use a summarization of your last interview with that person as the invitation. However, after your partner starts talking, limit yourself to either paraphrasing or summarizing your partner's content. If you want to ask a question to keep things moving, precede that question with a paraphrase or summarization. Stay immersed in his content, even if it is superficial. Superficiality of content is not the issue for this practice project; avoiding any focus on yourself is the issue, even to the point of not engaging in any sharing. These practice projects are not a simulation of what goes on in a real interview. They are exaggerations of what goes on during real interviews, with the purpose of refining a particular counseling skill. Once acquired, that skill would probably not be the only behavior you use, and would likely be timed and used differently or in conjunction with other behaviors in your interviews with your long-term interviewing partner.

There is also a negative practice approach to this practice project that could be helpful. It might sensitize you to any tendency you may have for injecting yourself inappropriately into the interview. Often, in conversations with friends, it is easy to fall into a "Can you top this" type of interaction. Your friend tells you something, and you may immediately think of something similar in your own experience and share it with him. This kind of thing can go back and forth several times. An easy example is joke telling. "Did you ever hear the one about. . . ." And you say "yes" or "no," listen to the joke, and come back with, "That reminds me of the one about . . ." and so on. This is part of the human experience. But it should not be a part of the counseling experience. Both negative and positive practice on this issue of absence of self-focus could be helpful.

No Noticeable Disinterest

Noticeable detachment and disinterest can quickly convey to the client that he, and what he is talking about, is not important enough to warrant attention by the counselor. In a sense, it is a rejection of the client by the counselor.

Unnoticeable Detachment

On the other hand, unnoticeable detachment in this circumstance is a positive attribute that suggests that the counselor remains neutral but attentive, without appearing aloof, indifferent, or disengaged from what is going on. What might constitute noticeable detachment or disinterest? Probably anything that the counselor might do that could compete with his attending behavior could be perceived as disinterest. Looking at your watch, or getting a book down from a shelf, while the client is talking, may be examples. Terminating eye contact, facing your chair away from the client, suggesting that the client talk about something else that is more important, even starting to fiddle with a paper clip or pencil, or doodling on a piece of paper—doing something that has nothing to do with what the client is currently doing or talking about can become a noticeable detachment or a show of disinterest. All of these things are risking a perception by the client that the counselor is not interested, and by their absence we mean that they should not be occurring and that the counselor should take care not to engage in them. Most of the time these things happen, not deliberately, but almost unconsciously, and the counselor has to be vigilant about his own behavior in this regard, or else he risks a weakening of the relationship.

SUGGESTED PRACTICE PROJECTS

Again in role playing and role switching, and with both positive practice and negative practice, you can enhance the development of this attribute of no noticeable detachment or disinterest.

From a positive perspective, an easy practice project is to engage in a great deal of verbal following during your practice interview with your short-term interviewing partner.

Merely echo (verbatim) the last word or few words that your partner said to you. This is a powerful way to communicate that you are interested and attending, almost without regard for any other types of disinterest you may be nonverbally showing.

A negative practice approach might involve your deliberately showing disinterest nonverbally as described earlier. When you do this type of thing intentionally, your awareness of the behavior, and your awareness of its consequences, should give you greater control over those behaviors, not merely through their inhibition, but through the behaviors that compete with them (e.g., echoing).

Ability to Tolerate Silence

The toleration of silence refers to the counselor's ability to tolerate both his own as well as the client's silence. Silence can have many functions for each of the participants. Silence by the counselor usually functions as an invitation to the client to talk. Sometimes, silence is combined with other nonverbal behaviors like head nodding, smiling, leaning forward toward the client, and sustained eye contact, to function as an encouragement for the client to continue talking. Sometimes the counselor is uncomfortable with his own silence because he thinks it may somehow convey to the client that he is incompetent, or doesn't know what to say, or know what direction the conversation should move toward. Some silence is intentional because it has an intentional function regarding the client. Sometimes it is because the counselor is thinking about what was just said, and such thoughtfulness during silence might be necessary and also perceived as necessary by both the counselor and the client.

For the client, his own silence can have functions that are similar to the ones just mentioned with regard to the counselor. The client may be inviting the counselor to talk, the client may not wish to talk, the client may be thinking about what the counselor has just said, or what he himself has just said. It is important for both parties to become comfortable with silence. It does not have to result in an awkwardness between the participants. Usually after 5 seconds of silence by the client, it is probable that he is not going to continue talking, and the counselor may wish to do something. He may openly acknowledge the silence and ask the client about it. He may in advance inform the client that silences may occur, and that they may or may not mean anything of significance. He can explain further, that when they do occur they aren't necessarily an embarrassment or awkwardness between them, and that they can explore them as they may come up during their time together, to understand them more fully.

SUGGESTED PRACTICE PROJECTS

Silence by either the counselor or the client is not a passive process. With your short-term practice partner during a practice interview, you can try various tactics for becoming comfortable with silence.

As the counselor in these practice circumstances you should certainly try to maintain your own silence while your partner is talking. This is a time for you to listen and attempt to understand what your partner is communicating to you. However, once your partner has become silent, try to maintain your silence for at least 10 seconds, thereby pushing your own toleration limits to the edge. Typically a client will talk within 5 seconds, if he is going to continue. But for practice purposes stretch it out to 10 seconds, both for extending your tolerance levels of silence, and to provide an extended opportunity for your partner to continue talking. But during this silence the counselor should be trying to figure out, if it is possible, what the function of this silent experience is for the partner. What does the partner want to have happen? Is he waiting for you talk? Is he thinking about something? After the 10-second interval, if the partner is still silent, then you can break the silence with whatever appropriate comment you wish to make.

If you wish, you can extend the mutual silence periods for longer intervals. Both of you may laugh, or feel uneasy, or comment about it. It can become a game of control and power, of who will talk first, or stay silent the longest. Don't avoid discussing any of this with your partner. Such a discussion of your mutual feelings about silence might prove to be helpful in dealing with future silent experiences with each other.

Avoidance of Superficial Content

Recognizing that clients may often drift away from talking about their problems, for any number of reasons, into superficialities, the counselor can employ a number of tactics to prevent that from occurring. Summarizing previous content themes that the client talked about, asking questions that are open but leading; in terms of circumstances, making comments that suggest or describe themes that may relate to themes already introduced by the client can be helpful in keeping out superficial content. Open invitations from the counselor to the client to talk, that carry with them the theme to be considered, such as "Tell me more about your family," tells the client the content area to explore. If the counselor thinks this is necessary from prior experiences with the client it is a less risky tactic.

On the other hand, we should not be too quick to engage in such leading tactics because it doesn't permit the client to set the thematic agenda, or to lead the counselor in his own way, with his own style, whatever it may be, into those areas that may be quite pertinent. When the counselor takes the lead in order to avoid superficiality he may shut off very pertinent areas of issues that might not otherwise become available for consideration. It is a tactic to be employed with much caution.

SUGGESTED PRACTICE PROJECTS

The role play and switching roles is also the vehicle for learning more about this tactic of avoiding superficial content.

In this instance, the short-term interviewing partner should be programmed for dwelling on superficial content, to provide the opportunity for the counselor to do something about it. The partner can choose to talk about anything that is unimportant, for example, the weather, the movies, TV, what to wear, what to eat, the latest news, things about other people, but nothing about himself. The counselor in turn can practice his attempts, as previously mentioned, to get the partner back into some meaningful content area.

From a different, negative practice perspective, the counselor can pick up on the partner's superficial content, and deliberately expand it, clarify it, encourage it through questions or minimal encouragers, to make him more sensitive to what he is deliberately doing that he doesn't want to do.

Appropriate Topic Change

There may be many times during a counseling session when the conversation drifts away into irrelevance, or is not on the target of content that was being developed. As the counselor tries to arrange for the client to set the agenda, the topics of conversation can range over a number of themes. One never knows early in a relationship how a person thinks, how his mind works, how he may associate one theme or topic to another. Sometimes a client has to "meander" through a number of themes in order to address what he is really after, almost like he is circling the terrain before mounting his attack on himself. It's almost as though he has to go through some indirect route, to create his own comfort level, or think through a series of associative events in some indirect detour to get to where he really wants to go. The counselor should let this happen so that the client can finally get to the point.

If it becomes blatantly clear that the commentary by the client is not going anywhere, or that the client has lost his train of thought or has forgotten where he was originally intending to go in his themes, then the counselor may try in a number of ways to get the client back onto a more relevant track. The counselor might merely say, "I'm not sure I'm following you." Or, if the counselor sees where the client was headed, he can take the lead to get him back into his commentary in the direction the counselor thinks he was headed, with a simple summary or paraphrase of what has just been said, but then adding the appropriate content that may have slipped away from the client.

On the other hand, if all of the client's commentary was quite irrelevant, he may either permit the client to complete his comments, and then say "That was interesting, but maybe you could help me see how that relates to what we were talking about before." Or the counselor might interrupt the client in order to save some time, saying almost the same thing that was just suggested. He might also say, without even referring to the client's irrelevant commentary, "I'd like to know more about what we were talking about before." Each of these are designed to get the client back into relevant content themes, to the topics that relate to his problems. But again, proceed with caution, because there are many verbal and emotional routes that people take in order to honestly address what's really on their minds.

SUGGESTED PRACTICE PROJECTS

The mutual role play, similar to the previous role play, would again be appropriate. The partner would be programmed to engage in superficial content during this interview as well.

In this instance the counselor, after an appropriate listening interval during which he becomes fairly certain that a topic change is in order, can become more proactive. This means becoming much more directive relative to topic selection, but tempering that directiveness with his reaching back for topics previously introduced by the client.

On some occasions, however, it may become blatantly obvious that certain themes have been omitted, such as discussion of certain members of the family, or not talking about his communication problem, or how he spends his spare time, etc. It could be quite appropriate to introduce such a topic, with a comment like "You've never mentioned your father during our meetings." Of course, practice in engaging in such maneuvers provides experience in working with the intentionality and focus that has been mentioned so often, and it also provides you with the experience of what the consequences of such an introduction might generate. Your partner might acquiesce and talk about that topic, or resist and refuse. It could open up an entirely new series of issues for consideration, and could be well worth experiencing some of the discomfort that may occur, as well as possibly postponing or enhancing new self-discoveries.

You can never be certain where being proactive will take you, and whether it will be helpful or destructive, and whether it erodes or enhances the relationship relative to who takes the lead. It is a judgment about one instance and is probably worth exploring, especially if it results in the partner learning from it.

Appropriately Reinforcing

This holistic attribute is designed to generate a general positive atmosphere to the interview. Remembering the dual roles of communication specialist plus counselor, there will be occasions when the counselor may find himself reinforcing the "speech performance" of the client as he utilizes the interview for speech practice purposes. If such verbal reinforcers are brief, they probably do not interfere with the process of counseling. Also, being intermittently supportive of the client does not necessarily have to be limited to the client's efforts relative to his speech.

Supportive comments by the counselor may relate to the client's efforts to act on issues that have come up relative to his relationships with people. The counselor may reinforce how the client feels about some issue that has been a problem in the past. The counselor may be supportive of any type of positive changes perceived by the counselor relative to the client's understanding of how he feels and how those feelings affect what the client does. The counselor may encourage the client to continue in some way of thinking, or exploring a particular issue, or even behaving (without the counselor initially suggesting these endeavors). Such encouragements could be very helpful and serve as powerful reinforcers for the client to continue something he is pursuing that could be helpful in the counseling sphere of his total therapeutic experience.

SUGGESTED PRACTICE PROJECTS

The method for practicing being "supportive" is through a mock interview with your short-term interviewing partner. After providing the appropriate invitations to talk, you might try to focus your client on some topic through paraphrasing content or reflecting feelings, and follow-up with letting him know how well he is doing in understanding, expressing, or talking about important things. Do not issue any positive judgments about the content itself, but rather about the process that he is engaging in; for example:

Counselor: "You have a good understanding of what you have to do in your outside practice activities."

You might also do this by summarizing some theme and tracing where he was to where the client is at that moment, and the progress he has made in acting on things that have been discussed. Such reinforcement in your real world might also include supportive comments about changes in his communication skills, speech, and language, but in this practice situation that would not be appropriate. However, if your partner has revealed any really intimate and personal material that was but no longer is stressful, you can be supportive of his actions in that regard; for example:

Counselor: "I'm glad that you feel comfortable enough to tell me about how you feel. It makes these practice interviews so much more meaningful."

Generates Warmth and Trust

This is another of those holistic attributes that can give you a more comprehensive and probably more accurate understanding if you inspect the entire interview. Many of the specific behaviors discussed earlier may relate to this, but in this instance we are not tabulating specifics (although this might be possible).

It is being suggested that you can perceive this attribute partly by the depth of the content of what the client talks about. You can tell if the client is "letting the counselor in" if he is talking about very private, possibly intimate details about himself. If the client is sharing his feelings, as well as talking about things that are generally not for everyone's ears, it is a sign that there is a warm and trusting relationship either developing or already in place.

Client: "It's amazing what has happened here. I feel like I can tell you about anything that's on my mind. And it helps me when I do that. Amazing, in such a short time, too."

If in your examination and analysis of the tape recordings of the interviews with your long-term interviewing partner you hear yourself sharing, then you might also think that the trust is a two-way street; that is, the counselor is also willing to trust the client with information about himself.

Another indicator is the occurrence of a confrontation from either party. Although it is thought that a confrontation is usually an aversive event, probably for both parties, the very fact that it is taking place—and its style of execution as well as the client's reaction to it—may be an indicator of how much trust is operating between the client and counselor.

Client: "You know, 2 weeks ago I couldn't have told you this. But when you told me that you were going through a lot of what I was experiencing, and actually told me about it, I knew I could trust you."

Also, the body language, the nonverbal communication, and the appropriate physical space (not too close but not so far away that you couldn't touch his arm) are important indicators of warmth and trust.

Finally, the paralinguistic properties of the speech of both the client and the counselor, and how well they possibly match each other in tone, loudness, and rate, may reflect the warmth and trust that prevails in the interview. We are referring here not to a close matching, but to a sensitivity by the counselor to be somewhere close to where the client is with regard to how fast he talks, how loud his voice is, and by emitting an accepting tone of understanding.

SUGGESTED PRACTICE PROJECT

There are no suggestions for ways to practice warmth and trust as such. It is an outgrowth of the many other behaviors and attributes that characterize the interview. If the nonholistic facilitative behaviors are operating and active, and the holistic facilitative attributes are present in the interview, then warmth and trust will also be an active part of the counseling interviews.

Tolerates Crying

Crying during an interview is not uncommon, but it doesn't occur frequently enough to warrant a regular tabulation of its occurrences. But when it does occur, it should be noted, as well as the circumstances that seem to be related to it, such as certain content themes or feelings.

Also, it usually is not characteristic of an entire interview. When crying occurs, it stands out, as does the counselor's reaction to it. Suffice it to say at this point that the counselor should not impede its occurrence, but rather permit the person to express this form of emotion. Because it is such a special kind of event and sometimes generates emotional and personal reactions in the counselor, it is discussed in a special section in chapter 9, with appropriate ways for generating opportunities for the counselor to deal with it.

During the interviews with your long-term interviewing partner, if it occurs it should not be discouraged. And if your own tears become a part of it, let that happen as well, because it may communicate your deep understanding of where your interviewing partner is at that moment, and that you are there with him.

Counselor: "It's all right to feel, especially with what you told me has been going on. Go ahead, it's OK. Let it out."

Tolerates Emotional Language

There are moments during interviews when a client gets very excited, sometimes in happiness, sometimes in anger. Sometimes during his feelings of hostility, self-pity, and even sadness, he may get very emotional, almost losing control by screaming and shouting. The language used to convey his thoughts and feelings may be full of what we commonly refer to as "four-letter words." Even though unacceptable in polite society, we should try to remember that they are only words. They are stated in the privacy and confidentiality of a counseling session. They may or may not be characteristic of the client outside of the interview. The counselor must not show any negative reactions to the specific words used even though you may dislike them. Being accepting means accepting almost anything that may be forthcoming from the client, short of physical violence to you and others in the session, short of hurting himself, and short of damage to your property. These are the ways that the client has available to communicate to you at that moment. It may even represent an abrupt switch in language that may have some significance for the client and the counselor. Everything that the client communicates has a potential for importance, and therefore the situation should be generally free-flowing and remain unjudged from a moral, spiritual, or cultural standpoint.

Counselor: "You don't have to apologize. I know that really got to you. I think that's the first time I ever heard you curse. If it helps, go ahead with it that way. Hell, we all have our moments."

SUGGESTED PRACTICE PROJECTS

The most valid way to determine your tolerance for emotionally loaded language, including the unacceptable four-letter words, is to listen to your tape recording of the interviews and see if your interviewing partner used them. If he did, what was your reaction to it? If such language was not singled out for any overt reaction by you, then you should try to remember, or determine when you hear it on the tape, whether you have any covert reactions to it. If not, then it is not an issue.

However, its acceptability may depend on the nature and theme and context of its usage.

If it has not occurred or has occurred too infrequently to enable you to decide, then a desensitization role-playing experience with your short-term interviewing partner might be helpful.

Each of you, independently, might jot down a list of words and phrases that are typically not used in polite society. Make two copies, and then rate them on a scale from 1 to 5, with 1 being totally unacceptable and 5 being totally acceptable. Jot down any other comments you might want to make about them, in terms of their context for usage, people involved, and so on. Then go through a desensitization session, whereby each of you uses the other person's rating list, starting with words and phrases having a rating of 5 (most acceptable), and progressing to words with a rating of 1 (least acceptable), saying the words on the other person's scaled list to that person. The listener should let you know if he is reacting. If he does react negatively, then he should repeat that phrase himself, until he realizes "They are only words," then go on progressing through the list.

If he still reacts negatively, then the reader might preface his use of each word or phrase with a statement such as "I am now going to say the word or phrase 'god-damn-it' to defuse the emotionality that might be connected to it."

This should be followed by conducting a short interview with your interviewing partner deliberately using these four-letter words periodically as they may crop up during an actual interview. Roles should be reversed so that each of you has the experience of saying and hearing these words, thereby enhancing your unemotional reactions when and if they do come up in an actual counseling session.

Given these operational definitions, suggested goals, and practice projects for these holistic, facilitating properties of the counseling interview, you can better understand your inspection of Table 10.1, which lists them and provides examples of each, as well as Table A.2 in Appendix A.

These holistic factors that characterize varying amounts or segments of the interview require ongoing evaluation. Appendix A includes an evaluation form with a rating scale that is to be used for evaluating your current status and for tracking changes in these attributes of your interviews.

Changes are not necessarily linear nor progressive. The presence or absence of these attributes may vary with things that you do during the interviews, with things that your interviewing partner does as a reaction to what you do, or as a result of outside influences on your partner that have very little to do with what you do during the interview. When you see abrupt changes in these attributes from one interview to the next, you should try to analyze what is going on and keep a written record of your thoughts about these changes, including documentation, if possible, from the interviews, to see if you can observe some evolving pattern.

TABLE 10.1
Facilitative Holistic Attributes of the Counselor

Attribute		*Example*
Client-centered	Counselor:	"It would be helpful if you tell me what it is about yourself that you want to change."
	Client:	"My speech."
	Counselor:	"What about your speech?"
Accepting	Client:	"I feel I can't handle all this, my husband's stroke, his speech, my job."
	Counselor:	"It's been hard for you, I can see that. And it doesn't seem fair that it's all falling on you."
Fluent	Counselor:	"You're asking some difficult questions. We don't have all the answers and we never really know how things are going to turn out when we first start. Let's see where we are."
Concerned and empathic	Counselor:	"It has to be frustrating to know that you didn't get that job because of the way you talk. Anyone would be angry."
Relaxed and calm	Counselor:	"You're facing a big decision. I know it's not easy to talk about it. But let's not rush into anything too quickly."
Does not interfere or impede	Counselor:	(Nonverbal, silent listening or head-nodding, maintaining good eye contact. Verbally he may briefly encourage the client by saying such things as "Yes," or "I see," or "uh-hum.")
Does not judge	Counselor:	"I know you've been wrestling with your guilt and your shame for quite awhile and you want to end all of that now. Talking about it can help."
Does not suggest or give answers	Counselor:	"I know you feel it would be easier for you if I told you what to do. I'll look at it with you, but you also know that only you can answer that for yourself."
Does not deny feelings	Counselor:	"What you're feeling, at this moment, this freedom and excitement, it's as powerful as your guilt over it. They're both a part of where you are right now."

(Continued)

TABLE 10.1
(Continued)

Attribute		*Example*
Absence of self-focus	Counselor:	"I know what you mean, that sense of freedom, like a weight has been lifted off of you. You feel like you really know yourself, where you've been, where you are, and maybe where you want to go."
No noticeable disinterest	Counselor:	(Nonverbal, attending, and appropriate eye contact. Verbal—staying on client's content.)
Tolerates silence	Counselor:	(Counselor remains silent; silence waiting for client response [at least 5 seconds] while maintaining eye contact.)
Avoids superficial content	Counselor:	After initial greetings, verbally directing client to appropriate content: "Have you thought about what we last talked about?"
Appropriate topic change	Counselor:	"What you've been talking about, your speech, is it related to how comfortable you feel when you talk on the phone, or order in a restaurant, or is it just when you talk to authority figures?"
Listens and attends	Counselor:	(Verbal and nonverbal, eye contact, body posture, nodding of head to show you understand, verbal encouragement to continue.)
Appropriately reinforcing	Counselor:	(Being verbally supportive for certain classes of responses relating to counseling and to speech mechanics.) "You've really taken a big step. I think you're moving in the right direction."
Generates warmth and trust	Counselor:	(Judged from tone of counselor's voice and content of client's topics.) "I understand how much she still means to you. I know this is hard for you to face."
Tolerates crying	Counselor:	(Being supportive, permitting crying to continue rather than trying to cut it off.) "It's all right to let it out. It can even help."
Tolerates emotional language	Counselor:	(Not reacting negatively to client's choice of words and feelings.) "I never heard you talk about your father like that before. You've been holding back. Get it out, just the way it feels."

11

NONFACILITATIVE HOLISTIC ATTRIBUTES OF THE CLINICAL INTERVIEW

Now let us look at some of the nonfacilitative attributes that may generally characterize a counselor's interviewing and counseling. These are listed in Table 11.1, again with examples (out of context) of the ways in which these attributes may manifest themselves during an interview, as well as in Table A.2 in Appendix A. But before going to Table 11.1, it may again be helpful to have some operational definitions and state the possible goals for not having these holistic attributes of the interview.

These are things that we may wish to discard from the counseling interview if we see that they are occurring in the counseling sessions. Hopefully, they might never appear in your interviews, but these definitions and examples will help us to recognize them and then to discard them.

Where appropriate, Suggested Practice Projects are provided.

There are times when "negative practice," or doing the things you know that you do not want to do, will enhance your recognition of their untimely and unwanted occurrence. It is thought that such recognition by you will therefore decrease the probability of their occurrence, and this in turn will have a positive effect on your attitude and behavior of intentionally engaging in the appropriate, competing behaviors (Dunlap, 1932).

When you engage in such negative practice exercises, it might be well to inform your interviewing partner what you are doing and why you are doing this during your brief mock interviews (to enhance your recognition of them so that you do not unintentionally engage in them).

You should not engage in such negative practice exercises during your interviews with your long-term interviewing partner. Hopefully, during these longer interviews you will reap the rewards of such practice activities, and they should be reflected in your weekly analysis of the tape recordings of these sessions, showing either a reduction or absence of the nonfacilitative factors.

Inattentive Posture

Inattentive posture refers to the counselor's space, his positioning of himself in relation to where the client might be sitting, and body movements. Examples are when the counselor is not facing the client, or creating too much space between the counselor and client, such as sitting a great distance away, staring out the window, and so on. The consequences of such postures and movements may be that the client may feel alone, even in the counselor's presence, does not feel valued by the counselor, does not feel important enough to warrant some type of closeness or engagement; or the client may feel a lack of interest and warmth from the counselor. Each of these inattentive postures and their potential consequences can have a negative effect on the development of a trusting relationship between the client and counselor, and can affect whether the client will confide any significant material to the counselor.

SUGGESTED PRACTICE PROJECT

During your brief 10-minute mock interviews with your short-term interviewing partner, deliberately engage in several of the nonfacilitative activities just mentioned, such as facing away and looking out the window, walking around the room, tapping a pencil, or looking at your watch. Do this both when your partner is talking and when you are talking. Afterwards, you might discuss the effects of these activities on your interviewing partner to further imprint on yourself the effects of such activities. You should then reverse roles so that you are the recipient of such tactics and have their effects further imprinted on you.

Gaze Averted

This refers to the counselor's gaze pattern, not the client's. The counselor is supposed to look at the client when the client is talking to him, and when he is talking to the client. But this kind of attentiveness should not be construed as staring. Obviously, staring at someone can make that person quite uncomfortable. There are times when looking away from the client may be appropriate, such as when the counselor is thinking about what the client just told him—and hopefully it is obvious to the client that is what is going on. Sometimes during silence the counselor's gaze pattern may go back and forth between direct eye contact and a momentary lack of eye contact, which may be quite appropriate and comfortable for both parties. But eye contact is a powerful indicator of listening and interest, and a continuing lack of eye contact could easily be misinterpreted as a lack of interest.

SUGGESTED PRACTICE PROJECTS

Again, negative practice during an interview with your short-term interviewing partner is the vehicle for deliberately engaging in doing what you know you do not want to do.

During the interview, as you listen and talk, deliberately engage in exaggerated gaze patterns. Close your eyes completely while listening as well as while talking to your partner. Turn your back to him during listening and talking. Intentionally look down at the floor while he is talking. Afterwards, again discuss the effects of these actions on him. Then reverse roles, so that you also experience the same effects.

Incongruent Affect

This holistic attribute refers to the presence of frequent instances when the feeling tone of the counselor, or the emotions of the counselor, are inappropriately out of sync with those of the client. Any type of emotional reactions revealed by the counselor during a counseling session are usually considered inappropriate. But in this instance we are referring to incongruent emotional reactions, whereby there is a blatant mismatch between what the client has revealed and the counselor's reaction, either in terms of not appreciating the significance of the client's feelings, or reacting with his own emotions that do not match the client's emotional reactions. For example, the client has been describing an event, such as the loss of a relationship and is quite sad about it. He has shown his sadness through his facial expressions and tone of voice, and the words to describe his feeling. It would be incongruent affect if the counselor smiled and said, "If only everyone could be as lucky you are that this happened this way. In its way it solved your problems." The counselor is showing a totally different emotional response through his rate of speech, volume, and tone as well as the content of what he said. It is incongruent with the experience of his client at that moment. In fact, this interpretation may even prove to be a valid one, but it is inappropriate at that point in time because of what the client is feeling at that moment. Such incongruence of affect between the client and the counselor communicates to the client that the counselor does not understand what the client feels, and undermines the client's confidence in the counselor. Such events are blatant and disappointing examples to the client that he and the counselor are not communicating well, or that the spin or interpretation offered by the counselor of what was just told to him by the client shows how far apart they are from each other in terms of empathy, understanding, and values.

SUGGESTED PRACTICE PROJECTS

Again, negative practice of the unwanted attribute can be effective. By intentionally exaggerating the attribute during a mock interview with your short-term interviewing partner, that unwanted attribute will stand out for you.

During your mock interview, deliberately demonstrate through your actions or comments that your response is out of sync with what your partner has been telling you. By laughing at something that is quite serious, or deliberately misunderstanding a feeling, or showing a feeling that is quite the opposite of what your partner has just revealed, or offering an interpretation of a feeling (e.g., "You say you are afraid, but I think you think it's downright funny"), you can demonstrate how inappropriate you are in your response. At some point, you should explain to your partner that you are doing this on purpose and in an exaggerated form to accentuate it for yourself.

You should reverse roles so that you also experience such inappropriateness. As with the previous nonfacilitative holistic attributes, these negative practice exercises should not be carried out in the interviews with your long-term interviewing partner. Instead, the effects of such practice exercises should be revealed in your analyses of the weekly tape recordings of your counseling sessions by virtue of the absence or reduction in the occurrences of these attributes in your weekly interviews.

Stereotypic Minimal Encouragers

This refers to the use of the same nonverbal and verbal minimal encouragers to talk offered by the counselor to the client so as to only minimally influence the content of what the client talks about, while yet encouraging him to continue talking, which can have a negative effect on the client.

Nodding and smiling over and over again while the client is talking makes the counselor seem less interested and less genuine. The counselor becomes a humorous "head-bobber" and a "yes-man" if he has combined the word "yes" with his head movement. The same thing is true for the constant repetition of the same phrase, such as "I see," "I see," "I see," after each utterance by the client. Not only is it boring, but it also becomes meaningless and eventually could lose its value as a minimal encourager to talk. These short phrases and forms of minimally encouraging a client to talk should deliberately be varied, and the counselor should exercise some vigilance and judgment that he does not automatically fall into such a habit. Saying "Yes," "I see," "I understand," "um-hum," "uh-huh" are just a few of the many verbal expressions that can be employed at various times and that would thereby prevent the loss of the function of some of them, and certainly have an effect on how the client views your functioning.

SUGGESTED PRACTICE PROJECTS

In your mock interview with your short-term interviewing partner you should intentionally use the same minimal encourager, repeatedly, to sustain his talkativeness. Do this for 5 minutes, saying, for example, the words "yes, uh-huh" again and again, using only that form of minimal encourager. After 5 minutes, you can then switch to another one, such as "I see," and use that one for the next 5 minutes, limiting yourself to just those words as a form of encouraging your partner's talkativeness.

Reverse roles so that each of you has the experience of such a repeated tactic. It is not only boring to the listener, but it can become a distraction away from the topic of conversation. It can also communicate to the partner that you aren't really listening. This type of practice exercise should be limited to the short mock interviews with your short-term interviewing partner and should not be used in your weekly interviews with your long-term interviewing partner.

Questioning Impedes/Affects Agenda

The questioning by the counselor can either facilitate, affect, or impede the agenda. When this happens, it is usually not by design but by accident or unconsciously.

There are typically three forms of questions that do this, and they should be eliminated from the counselor's repertoire. One method of inappropriately questioning the client is by interrupting the client. The question may be relevant, but poorly timed because it abruptly changes the flow of talking by the client into a direction defined by the counselor. We often see this kind of event in many nonprofessional, interpersonal conversations when the listener is so eager and interested in what is being talked about that they interject their question while the speaker is still speaking. When an interrupter does this often, he eventually will be looked on in some negative way, as rude, only interested in his own opinions, or not listening, Most of the time, however, if it is only an occasional occurrence, the person gets away with it without any damage to his reputation as a conversational partner. But in counseling, it shouldn't happen even occasionally.

The second form of an impeding type of question that affects the agenda is again a timing issue. If a leading question that tells the client exactly what content the counselor wants to hear is asked very early in the interview, it is probably inappropriate because it not only directs the client into a specific content area, but also deprives the client of the opportunity to tell his story his way. For example, if the counselor says to the client, "Why don't we start with your family. What do you remember about your childhood?" it could shut down many other areas that may be on the client's mind that could be of greater significance, or that could help the client give a more comprehensive view of what he thinks is important and what he feels about the issues.

Interviews can be fact finding and information gathering, but they can also permit the client to take the lead. If specific areas of content are not covered in this open manner, the counselor can then ask his leading questions, and it would then be appropriate.

A third type of question that affects not only the agenda, but also affects how the client may answer a question, is one which tells the client what answer is being looked for. In other words, the answer is in the question. For example, if the counselor asks, "You say you lived at home. Did your parents do what most parents do, still treat you like a child and interfere with your relationships?" This question blatantly suggests an answer that the counselor would be sympathetic toward. A more open and less suggesting question might be, "What was it like, living at home after being away at college?" Although even this question suggests that there may have been a difference between living at home before and after college, it is much less suggestible regarding the nature of those differences.

SUGGESTED PRACTICE PROJECTS

With the method, assumptions, and goals of negative practice, you can intentionally ask questions that impede or affect content.

However, as a first step toward seeing both the negative and the positive aspects of asking leading questions, you might want to quickly examine most intake questionnaires that new patients and clients have to fill out on the occasion of their first visit to a professional office. The questions or instructions for responses are typically quite leading, and specifically tell you what categories of information are being sought. Although they do tap into what the staff feels is the most significant information they need to get started with your diagnosis or treatment (especially in medical situations), the questions typically do not provide the immediate freedom for the client to get into those things that they think may be of uppermost significance. Such questionnaires have their place and value in certain situations, especially if the client is provided an opportunity later to freely express his concerns as he experiences them.

Such an examination of that type of questionnaire will accentuate for you the leading nature of such questions and instructions. This should then be followed up with the negative practice experience of deliberately asking closed questions, leading questions, and questions that contain answers.

This latter type of question, containing a desired answer, should be focused on because it can occur so often, quite by accident and without any awareness that it has occurred.

Again, roles should be reversed with your partner. This type of practice also should not be employed with your long-term interviewing partner during your weekly interviews.

Denies or Doesn't Reflect Feelings

Much of counseling is helping the client focus on how he feels, helping him to understand his feelings, and acting on those understandings. If the counselor doesn't help him focus by reflecting the client's feelings back to him, that focus and understanding may be seriously retarded or never accomplished.

Losing an opportunity to reflect a client's feeling has the effect of denying its existence insofar as client self-discovery and focus is concerned.

Another form of denial occurs when the counselor tells the client that he "shouldn't feel that way" about something. Yet another form is to tell the client how he should feel, instead of reflecting how he currently feels.

Making a mistake by mislabeling a feeling is not a denial of feeling, and such mistakes can occur. It should not deter the counselor from continuing to reflect his client's feelings, but he should try to improve his accuracy. A high frequency of mislabeling can lead the client to feel that he and the counselor are not communicating, and that he is not being understood. This can damage the relationship, and erode the client's confidence in the competence of the counselor.

SUGGESTED PRACTICE PROJECTS

There are several ways to deny a client's feelings, and it might be well to become sensitive to each of them because you might find that your skills in reflecting feelings can coexist with occurrences of denying or rejecting feelings. Through the method of negative practice it is suggested that you deliberately inject such occurrences into your brief interviews with your short-term interviewing partner.

You can do this by looking for those occasions when your partner has revealed some type of feeling to you, and your response is one of "you shouldn't feel that way," or "don't worry, time will heal, and the feeling will go away."

On some other occasions of emotional expressions by your partner you might paraphrase the content, and totally ignore the feeling aspect of what was told to you.

On yet other occasions, in order to check on your accuracy of reflecting a feeling, you might ask your partner to affirm or correct, if need be, your reflecting of feeling. Each of these exercises should improve your skills in feeling reflection, and make you more sensitive to "missed opportunities" that may be occurring without your awareness.

Lengthy Response

This attribute refers to a consistent pattern by the counselor of commenting for too long a time.

Invitations to talk, comments that function to focus on a particular portion of the client's comments, as well as sharing and interpretations by the counselor, should be brief. This is not an interview that is designed to bring out the counselor's value system or point of view. Lengthy responses by the counselor suggest that the focus is more on the counselor than the client, and possibly that the counselor is "using" the client as a vehicle for focusing on himself. Also, the client is capable of processing just so much from the counselor. A multithemed comment by the counselor that would probably also be a long response will get lost in the myriad things that may be on the client's mind. Comments should be brief and easy to understand. If you find your self saying something like, "Let me try to explain that to you again," or "Wait, let me simplify what I just said," you should check yourself for both length and simplicity against the client's statements, as well as against your other comments when you didn't have to qualify what you just said to the client. Also, the more the counselor talks, the less the client talks, and as a result some of the goals of the counseling process are jeopardized, such as self-discovery and self-actualization.

Given what has just been said about length and complexity of response, there are occasions when the counselor's response will of necessity be longer than some of his other responses. This is especially true for the tactic of interpretation, when the counselor is telling the client something new that he feels would be helpful to the client if he knew it. It might be an explanation of cause and effect, or a perception of some type of relationship between events that the client has brought up. This type of comment will take longer to get across, but it still should remain simple and understandable.

SUGGESTED PRACTICE PROJECTS

There are several ways to engage in practice activities that reduce the likelihood of making responses that are too long. One of these is to alert your partner during your mock interview with him that after each paraphrase, feeling reflection, summarization, sharing, and interpretation, you are going to repeat, but shorten it, perhaps cut it in half. Then shorten it a second time and a third time, so that it is perhaps one or two phrases in length, and limited to a single and most significant theme. Discuss the result with your partner to see if it seems better when it is shorter, and how it is better. You should reverse roles so that you are also on the receiving end of such an exercise.

Self-Focus

This undesirable holistic attribute of the counselor during an interview means that the counselor is in the middle of the action far too much. The counselor inserts himself as the topic for attention, thereby reducing the focus on the client. This becomes evident when it's obvious that the counselor talks about himself too much, about his experiences, his feelings, his opinions, or what he values. He may use the client's comments as the vehicle for getting the attention focused on himself. Sometimes this occurs through interruptions by the counselor, as though the counselor was impatient or just couldn't wait to get his comments out on the floor between them. Sometimes this self-focus by the counselor is revealed by overly emotional reactions by the counselor, which focus on the counselor and not on the client. The judgmentalness by the counselor of the client's comments is yet another way that self-focus is shown. It almost seems as though the relationship has become more of a mutual conversation, much like our interpersonal conversations with friends, rather than a counseling session, wherein the conversational partners are exchanging information about themselves with each other, or playing "can you top this." Another way of characterizing selffocus is that the counselor has failed to subordinate himself in the counseling process. This self-focus can be very damaging to the client for a number of reasons. Focus on the client (and not on the counselor) carries with it a "role" to be played by each of the participants. The client learns what his role is in terms of self-responsibility, taking risks, taking the lead, for self-discovery and self-actualization. The client learns his own role from the counselor showing him the counselor's role. All of the aforementioned learning by the client will be jeopardized if the counselor does not function appropriately in his role of being subordinate to the client, and focusing on the client.

SUGGESTED PRACTICE PROJECTS

Loss of focus that is characterized by self-focus on the part of the counselor is one of the most disastrous nonfacilitative attributes one can encounter in a counseling session. Focus on the client is one of the building blocks that supports many of the other facilitative processes that occur in counseling. This type of problem can happen quickly, frequently, and almost unconsciously. Your awareness of self-focus is essential. This can also coexist with focus during a session. One moment you are totally focused on what your partner or client is saying, doing, or feeling, and the next moment you can be into yourself, focused on yourself, how you feel, your history, and your problems. Sometimes it is covert, and not verbally injected into the session, but it is there all the same in terms of what you are thinking about and what you are feeling. These personal reactions compete with your focus on your client, and ultimately can become so powerful that you become disengaged from your client, from his issues of concern, and from his reasons for being there with you. In your mind and thoughts, even though it may be for a brief period of time, you become the topic of your own focus.

It comes out in the form of talking about yourself and not about your client. A simple analysis of "talking time" can be very revealing. If the counselor is dominating the talking time with his own talking, then for one reason or another, the focus is on himself, perhaps as the "necessary interpreter" or "needed healer," or "directive advice giver," or the "revered and respected role model," thereby risking overdependence in his client.

Again, negative practice in the form of talking about yourself, warning your partner before you engage in it, to the point of exaggeration, can impress this type of behavior on you. Engage in such self-focus for long segments of time during a mock interview with your short-term interviewing partner, and then reverse roles with him so that you also experience the effects of such behavior. It can ruin a relationship. Experiencing both ends of this type of attribute should make you all the more wary, and enhance your prevention of it from occurring even accidentally.

Inappropriate Topic Change

The counselor is constantly making decisions during the interview, while the client is talking, during the silence of both participants, and even during his own comments, as to whether they are moving in the right directions, and talking about things that will eventually be helpful to the client. There will be occasions when the counselor takes the lead and changes the topic that is being discussed. The appropriate change of topics by the counselor is a cautious, deliberate, well-thought-out action. It leads the client into another theme that the counselor deems to be more helpful than the one the client is pursuing. If the counselor does this, he might well take his cues from what the client was talking about at some earlier time, if not the client's current commentary. In other words, the selection of topics should not be solely determined by the counselor; but if the counselor takes the lead into a topic, it should somehow be related to content themes that the client had previously addressed.

At times the counselor may want to take the client into an area of discussion that has never been brought up before. This could be appropriate if, after a time during the interview, the counselor has heard some things that he correlates or understands and may wish to make an interpretation of to the client. By definition, an interpretation is "new information" that the client might benefit from hearing from the counselor. However, usually such information is based on previously introduced comments, and such prior comments might well be summarized as a prologue to such interpretations. In such a summary, the content would not be an inappropriate change because it was already familiar, even though it might not relate to the immediately preceding comments of the client.

Inappropriate topic change refers to the abrupt change by the counselor of the content that was being discussed, especially if it does not seem to relate to anything that the client has talked about. It is also inappropriate if the counselor jumps in and changes topics without giving the client an opportunity to meander through his verbalizations about pertinent areas of discussion.

One of the possible consequences of such behavior by the counselor is that the client can become dependent on the counselor to take the lead in setting the agenda, become more passive in his demeanor, and engage in less risk taking and less self-discovery.

SUGGESTED PRACTICE PROJECTS

The use of negative practice to recognize when you do things that you know you don't want to do can accentuate their inappropriateness. By doing those things in an exaggerated way, you can sometimes further enhance your recognition of their occurrence. This would be the case for the negative practice of inappropriate topic change.

With your short-term interviewing partner during a short mock interview of 10 or 15 minutes, deliberately insert questions that are not related in any way to the material that your partner just talked about. In addition, you can issue open invitations to talk where you provide another topic than the one that was under discussion. They might even be comments that have a personal twist to them, such as "I just noticed your hair. Who is your barber? Where do you get your hair cut?" Obviously, such questions would have nothing to do with anything of pertinence or significance to your counseling session.

You should then reverse roles so that you also have the experience of being on the receiving end of such tactics.

Reinforces Superficial Content

When the client is engaging in making comments that are obviously superficial, the best thing that the counselor can do is to keep quiet, even though his silence may be interpreted by the client as an invitation to continue. Silence by the counselor is probably the most passive of his invitations to talk. Using such minimal action, the counselor is still permitting the client the opportunity to work his way through such superficialities into pertinence and all of the other possible helpful things that can happen when the client accomplishes such a journey.

The counselor should not actively try to weaken such superficiality by the client through various showings of disinterest. Instead, he should stay engaged and show his interest in the client—if not in the things he may be talking about—by maintaining good eye contact. But, at the same time, he might refrain from providing verbal invitations, minimal encouragers, questions, and echoing the endings of client comments, as though he wanted the client to continue in this vein. Hopefully, the client will eventually on his own, in the absence of counselor encouragement and possibly with the advent of his own and the counselor's silence, reach a point where he becomes aware that something is amiss. If the counselor provides such invitations and encouragers, he may well be unaware that he is reinforcing these superficial comments by the client. This often happens when the counselor is uncomfortable with silence and wants to keep the client talking without regard for the pertinence of the material.

Sometimes the counselor's stereotypical minimal encouragers, like nodding his head or saying "uh-huh" or "yes" may have become so automatic that he continues to provide them to the client without thinking about what he is doing. However, it is well to remember that it can be difficult to judge the superficiality of a comment or a series of comments immediately, or to judge the possible function of a series of comments as an aid to the client to move himself into content themes that may have greater significance in relation to his problems. It also may take some time to judge the possible avoidance function of superficiality, which in itself may be an appropriate topic for discussion and understanding by the client.

SUGGESTED PRACTICE PROJECTS

During your interview with your short-term interviewing partner you can approach negative practice of this attribute of reinforcing superficial content in several ways.

One way is for you to deliberately start your interview with some small chitchat about the weather, a TV show you saw, or how good the lunches are in the cafeteria, and try to stay on that topic. If your partner picks up on one of these themes, you can deliberately reinforce him by your various attending and listening tactics, your echoing of the last few words, by open and closed questions on the topic, even by reflecting his feelings about the topic. This intentional use of legitimate counseling tactics around superficial topics should alert you to how effective these tactics are, as well as accentuate your awareness of this particular kind of misuse. Your partner may passively resist, or make a comment, or ask you why you and he are talking about such superficialities. A truthful explanation regarding your need to negatively practice this type of interaction would be in order, followed by a suggestion that you switch roles so that each of you experiences it.

A second approach to this type of exercise is to interview your partner and merely wait for him to introduce some superficial material, which you would then intentionally reinforce in the same style and with the same tactics just mentioned.

If you recognize the content as superficial, you might also practice getting out of it by questioning its relevance, or indicating that you don't understand how it relates to the relevant material that was just discussed.

Shows Disrespect

The showing of disrespect for the client obviously has no place, nor justification, during the counseling process.

There will be many times when the client is revealing things to the counselor that may be aversive to the counselor. Anything that might collide with the counselor's values, beliefs, and spirituality, may generate a lack of respect from the counselor. However, even in the presence of such aversiveness, the counselor's job is to maintain a focus on what is going on in the world of the client. The counselor should try to understand what may have brought the client to such a condition, and how he can be helpful to the client regarding living with his current state of affairs or in making changes.

Such things as the client's racial, ethnic, and religious bigotry, confessions of verbal abuse, revealing his homosexuality, discussing his history of violence, his lack of regard for the law, or lack of respect for the rules of society, his politics, or attitudes toward certain politicians, may be issues that collide with the counselor's views about these things. The counselor should know himself and what he believes in, and be able to recognize the potential for various themes to generate such disrespect in himself for the client.

Such disrespect often contains elements of hostility and confrontation, sometimes even aggressiveness and anger by the counselor. Also, these negative feelings about the material that the client has revealed are often not separated from the client, and can be perceived by the client as being negative feelings about the client. Therefore, the client—as well as what he has revealed—can be perceived as the target of this disrespect. And it may well be that such disrespect for the client is actually the case.

But in all situations, the counselor has to keep himself under control, no matter how disgusting the material is that the client entrusts to him. He has to keep his focus on the client, and try to understand where he is coming from and how he can help him.

SUGGESTED PRACTICE PROJECTS

The first step in dealing with disrespect for the client would be to listen to the tape recordings of your counseling sessions with your long-term interviewing partner. If you identify anything that you think could be construed as disrespect for the person being interviewed, try to analyze what it might be related to, in terms of the themes being discussed. You may be able to identify some content area or something about him that bothers you.

Then, during your interview with your short-term interviewing partner ask him to bombard you with similar material so that you can get used to hearing it, while still maintaining your focus on him. This type of desensitizing, followed by your engaging in competing helpful counseling tactics, can do a lot to defuse any potential for disrespect by you.

You can also ask your partner to talk to you about any occasion when he may have noticed that you were disrespectful, and discuss the form that it took as well as the reasons for it.

You could take your practice a step further and warn your partner in advance that you were going to intentionally introduce some different forms of disrespect so that you can become more aware of this attribute, or become more aware of the first signs in yourself, such as a reaction to some specific content, that could lead to such behavior.

So that you can appreciate what your client or partner experiences as a reaction to disrespect, you should switch roles, and learn it firsthand. It is generally a very destructive and negative experience that can have long-standing consequences.

Shows Discomfort

When the counselor shows discomfort with the client or with what the client has revealed to him, he is again faced with the same challenge to maintain his focus on the client. Although this is not the same emotional condition as disrespect, the erosion of his focus is the same, perhaps without the element of hostility. The same cautions about the thematic content prevail, and the same sense of oneself and control of his feelings by the counselor is required. The counselor might do well to closely examine the entire interview to determine how often his negative emotional reactions are inserted into the interview.

If the counselor's reactions become holistic, or are characteristic of major portions of the interview, or are characteristic around certain themes, he might question whether he is the appropriate person to be counseling this particular client.

If things get to this point, the counselor might then wish to discuss these issues with a colleague or a supervisor in order to resolve this problem. Sometimes such discussions of the counselor's problems with being uncomfortable with his client are simple to resolve.

There may be some occasions and issues that are difficult for the counselor, regarding not only his focus, but also client confidentiality. If, in the process of the client's revelations, the counselor becomes aware of criminal intent or a criminal history of the client, it may be incumbent on him to inform the legal authorities that such is the case. The law requires such reporting, mostly in order to prevent a crime from occurring, or to prevent the client from hurting someone or hurting himself. If the counselor has any questions about the legal or ethical aspects of what has been revealed to him, he should immediately read through his professional code of ethics. If questions still remain in his mind about legal or ethical considerations of what the client shared with him, he would do well to contact his professional board of ethical practices. It might also be helpful to contact an attorney who has experience with such issues as professional ethics, client confidentiality, and the legal responsibilities of the counselor regarding the criminal acts of a client. Sometimes this may not be a clear-cut issue, and can be a severe test of the counselor's ethics versus adherence to the law.

If these revelations are violations of laws that the counselor thinks are unfair, perhaps as in substance abuse, especially if the counselor is counseling someone regarding such abuse, the lines of appropriate action can become very fuzzy. This is not an improbable circumstance. A person who has a communication problem will occasionally resort to drugs as a way of escaping from the realities of his communication problems.

However, the client confidentiality/legal/ethical issues are somewhat different from the problem referred to earlier of the counselor being personally antagonistic and uncomfortable with the content of what the client was revealing. The resolution is not an attempt to change the counselor's attitudes about that content. Rather, it is a problem of client focus, and the counselor being able to subordinate himself and his feelings at that time during a professional counseling interview, with specific attention to the thematic content that seems to generate the counselor's reactions. It is hard for the counselor to be a helpful facilitator if he is struggling with his own emotional reactions and ambivalence about the material in front of him during an interview.

If such uncomfortable reactions continue for too long a time it could well jeopardize the many things he has been trying to accomplish with that client. It could even mean referring that client to another counselor if this type of problem persists.

There is a general principle that emerges here for the counselor. One should not undertake counseling around certain problems if the counselor himself is experiencing similar problems that are as yet unresolved. This is also true if the counselor's reactions to certain content themes persistently interfere with his being helpful.

SUGGESTED PRACTICE PROJECTS

A process of role playing and desensitization with a colleague or training partner around those negative content themes may be helpful, such as having a partner deliberately introduce troublesome themes, again and again, and having the counselor maintain his focus by engaging in helpful interviewing tactics in the face of these content themes.

Is Judgmental

Passing judgment, moralizing, and giving approval or disapproval can have the effect of inhibiting the client.

Although the client may want the counselor's judgments, he generally wants only the positive ones, the ones that seem to agree with the client's self-judgments. If approval has been forthcoming in the past, the client can come to expect such approval in the future. When it is not forthcoming in the future, the client can easily assume disapproval by the counselor. Counseling is not a matter of "right" and "wrong" or "good" and "bad," but it can be a matter of "destructive" and "helpful" to the client in terms of what he is trying to make of his life. If the client perceives the counselor as generally disapproving, he may not examine and talk about those things that he himself feels guilty about or ashamed of in his past, or present ways of coping with his problems. Examining such intimate and personal issues with a counselor requires a trust that makes the client feel that he will not be judged or punished for his beliefs, feelings, and actions. It is only then that the client becomes willing to look at himself and be honest about himself.

Even in the tactic of confrontation, which by definition is aversive, there should be no judgment or punitiveness. Rather, it should be an honest mirroring or reflection of issues already introduced by the client that are not judged. Such content, instead, becomes appropriate for examination, understanding, and resolution. In this way, the counselor's honesty and persistence can become a model for such nonjudgmental examination, without moralizing about the issue.

However, if the client introduces his own morals as an issue, it should not be ignored. He may be violating his own sense of what is right and what is wrong, and as a result, make judgments about himself and feel guilty. The counselor's job is to help the client examine and deal with his own moralizing and self-judgments, and not introduce his own views or judgments about the issues. For example, a husband may be feeling guilty about separating from his wife because he feels it is wrong for him to do this after so many years of marriage. You as the counselor may privately agree or disagree with his moral judgment, but it is the client who has to resolve this issue for himself in terms of his own comfort and feelings about himself. You can help him examine these issues, help him to get in touch with his feelings under various circumstances of his past and present, as well as his speculations about his future; but the ultimate decision is his, without the influences of your belief system.

SUGGESTED PRACTICE PROJECTS

Judgmentalness in an interview that involves both speech therapy and counseling happens in many different ways and in many different forms. Often, the client seeks your judgment as a speech pathologist, and it may be entirely appropriate for you to share your judgment with him about issues involving his communication problem. These might include the value of tactics for therapy, and how he arranges to practice his new skills that focus on his communication problem.

But he may also seek your judgment on things other than his communication problem. They might be related to his communication problem, or unrelated to it, where your sharing of your judgment could deprive him of the opportunity to independently discover and explore various issues about himself. As ironic as it may seem, they may deal with problems that are generated by the progress he is making in dealing with his communication problem. There are long-standing relationships with loved ones that may have changed because of the positive changes in the client's speech. There may be new expectations for himself and for his family, a new self-concept, or the experience of giving up the secondary rewards of his problem—such as his helplessness or having an excuse for failures that both he and his family are learning to live with. The point is that the client may be seeking your approval and judgment about many different kinds of issues, and your approval constitutes a judgment by you.

If you agree with the idea that one of the goals of counseling is to have your client eventually operate from a perspective of internal locus of control, then his dependence on your judgments defeats that purpose.

In addition, the counselor may inadvertently make judgments that are not being sought by the client. The counselor may have had many experiences in his life that are similar to those of his client, and therefore he may have a position, attitude, or opinion about these issues that he feels puts him in a unique position to judge the correctness of what his client thinks, feels, and does in relation to these similar issues. This can be an issue for speech therapists, wherein the therapist may have had a speech problem much like that of his client, and feels that his own experiences, attitudes, feelings, and resolutions would be appropriate for his client. Or the counselor may have other things in common with his client such as being married, or divorced, or being a parent, or an only child, that he believes gives him the privilege to judge his client's feelings and actions because of their similar histories.

You should try to determine whether you have a tendency to share your opinions and beliefs. You can find that out by examining the tape recordings of your interviews with your long-term interviewing partner, or you may already know this about yourself from your interpersonal interactions with friends and relatives. If you do have this tendency, then practice projects on this subject are critical.

Try to practice separating being supportive from being judgmental. An example is that it is appropriate to encourage your partner's willingness to share some personal information, and to let him know that you appreciate how difficult that can be, and how courageous he is in trusting you and taking such risks, without necessarily condoning or approving the content of what he tells you. In other words, you can say "I understand" without saying "That's great," or "Wow."

Do not evaluate the validity of what he tells you. Accept it. If you don't believe it, tell him that you don't understand what he just told you, or ask him to explain it more clearly. Don't say "I find that hard to believe." These are evaluative judgments that could ruin a relationship and inhibit his sharing for fear of your judgments. This can be done in your interviews with your short-term interviewing partner, and also with your long-term partner. Switch roles again with your short-term partner so that you experience it from the interviewee's standpoint.

Gives Advice

It seems altogether appropriate for the speech clinician to give information and guidance about how to change or improve communication. Giving advice about how to execute a particular maneuver relative to speaking may be essential and required for the learning of new speech behaviors. This is certainly part of the speech pathologist's job. This may also extend into how the client may organize his transferring of these new skills into his everyday life away from the clinician.

However, the client should be encouraged to develop some of those ideas for himself if he is ever going to be free of his need for therapy or for the therapist.

Dealing with the impact of change should require a major and leading role for the client. He should be encouraged to organize his strategies as he is comfortable with them. Changing the way you talk commonly involves changing the way you see yourself as a person. There can be new expectations, new stresses, changing the nature of relationships, becoming independent, and giving up the many secondary rewards that may be associated with having a communication problem. The client must decide to set the agenda for integrating his new communication skills into his life.

The client may decide to take things as they come, and adopt a reactive style, which may have been the way he did things in the past. Or, he may decide to adopt a proactive style, to take risks, educationally, occupationally and socially, and in his interpersonal relationships. These are his decisions. He has a right and a need to make them, a right to experience his life as he wishes. Even when you, as his speech therapist and as his counselor, feel that he might be making things harder for himself than is necessary or that he might be going down the wrong road (the road you wouldn't choose for yourself!), we must remember that he has a right to do it his way, to experience it his way, and possibly to learn from it. That is the way he will learn. Without your advice, he has an opportunity to develop an internal locus of control, and an opportunity to develop an internal system for evaluating what he is about. Hopefully, he will learn how to revise what he is believing, feeling, and doing, if he so wishes. Your advice giving could retard all of that significant learning that may lie ahead of him. Your advice may be a shortcut for him, and might possibly make things easier for him, but your eagerness to be helpful could cut out of his experience what he may need most: to be free and independent in learning to make decisions for himself.

SUGGESTED PRACTICE PROJECTS

Listen to your tapes and determine if you have been giving advice. You will also know this from your weekly evaluations of your interviews with your long-term interviewing partner. But your easiest source of recognition is what you do with your friends. Your personal interactions are often a good predictor for how you might behave during counseling interviews, that is, until you become aware of and recognize what you are doing.

Negative practice, or intentionally giving advice in an exaggerated manner to your short-term interviewing partner during a short interview on just about everything he talks to you about, will get both of you to recognize its occurrence very quickly. This can be done, almost humorously, on insignificant topics, like what clothes to wear, what and where to eat, when to go to sleep. In a sense, you are telling him how to live out his daily routine. Then reverse roles so that each of you experiences receiving advice. Its exaggeration in type and frequency will enhance your negative awareness of its occurrence, and should probably prevent it from occurring during your counseling interviews with your long-term interviewing partner, and it may even carry over into some of your interpersonal interactions.

Interrupts

Interruptions by the counselor have already been discussed. It is the one type of behavior that is very close to becoming a "thou shalt not" axiom. The counselor always has an opportunity to insert his comments during an interview. Sometimes the counselor's interruption is a function of his overeagerness to insert his comment, without regard for its timeliness or its consequence. Sometimes the interruption has more to do with the counselor than with the client, and may be an instance of the counselor losing his focus on the client. However, most often an interruption by the counselor is made because he thinks his comment would be more helpful than a continuation or completion of a thought by the client. This may well be true, and on those occasions it would be appropriate for the counselor to interrupt in order to terminate superficial content. But there is always the risk that the interruption will detour the client away from some material that he is using to ready himself for revealing more significant material to the counselor.

The counselor should not be rude or disrespectful if he interrupts, but should wait for his opportunity. Even then, the counselor must decide if it is worth the risks of what this may do to the client, knowing that his chance to comment will eventually arrive.

SUGGESTED PRACTICE PROJECTS

Again, your practice exercises on interruptions should be preceded by an examination of your interpersonal interactions with friends (Do you interrupt when talking to your friends?), as well as an analysis of your tapes of prior sessions with your long-term interviewing partner. You should find out if this is one of your weak points—a tendency not to let your conversational partner finish his utterance.

The most effective way to practice this is to do it on purpose, and again with an exaggerated frequency. During a brief interview with your short-term interviewing partner, jump in before he can finish, sometimes even at the beginning of his utterance. Enduring this is more than just a nuisance probably for you as well as your partner.

Do this during a 5-minute interview. Then reverse roles so that you are on the receiving end to experience this aversive type of dyadic conversation.

Inappropriate Confrontation

Confrontations by the counselor can have a powerful impact on the client in several ways. By definition it has some aversive properties to it, and the counselor has to be careful that these aversive elements are not expressed in any judgmental or punitive form. Usually the function of a confrontation is that it is a "wake-up call" for the client to understand something about himself that he currently misunderstands. It may have come out as a self-contradiction by the client, or faulty reasoning, or a process of denial or rationalizing and finding excuses. It may involve his exploiting his communication handicap to generate secondary rewards for himself. Whatever the content of the confrontation may be, the counselor must be gentle but firm. The counselor not only communicates the content of his confrontation but also his honesty, tenacity, and understanding, which could function as a model for the client to engage in self-confrontation.

SUGGESTED PRACTICE PROJECTS

With your short-term interviewing partner during a 10-minute interview, develop a generally confrontational attitude. Question, in a negative way, just about everything he tells you. Ask him, "How do you know that?" after he has told you something. Or, without judgment, state, "That really doesn't sound like you." Continue this throughout the 10 minutes. Then reverse roles so that it becomes a shared experience.

Inappropriate Sharing

When the counselor shares something from his own experience, he supposedly does it as a tactic to help the client in several different ways. It communicates to the client that the counselor understands, that the client is not the only one who might have experienced a similar problem, that the client is not alone, but has an understanding companion, and that the counselor is willing to take the same risks as the client by entrusting the client with confidential material about himself or herself. It can also be helpful as a vehicle for clarifying some similar issue for the client. The challenge for the counselor is to be able to be brief, to share a portion of his own experience that relates to the feelings and/or circumstances that are troublesome to the client, with very little focus on the counselor's commentary. It should be worded in such a way that the client easily sees that the counselor's commentary, although about himself, still retains a focus on the client, and is really about the client.

It is inappropriate sharing if it is too long, takes up too much talking time, is off target relative to the client's problems, doesn't match up with the significance of the client's problems, or develops a focus by the client or the counselor on the counselor's experience. It is also inappropriate if the counselor's comments suggest an answer or give advice, or relate how he, the counselor, resolved his problem.

If any of these elements of inappropriate sharing are present, the consequences can take many negative or nonhelpful forms. They can communicate to the client that the counselor is not listening, is only thinking about himself, or doesn't understand what the client is experiencing, and could deprive the client of an opportunity to experience the process of self-discovery and the freedom to resolve an issue on his own without the intervention and advice of the counselor.

SUGGESTED PRACTICE PROJECTS

The key to the appropriateness of sharing is timing and matching. You should examine your interviews with your long-term partner to determine if you have done any sharing at all, whether it was introduced into the interview in relationship to something that your partner was talking about, and whether it matched your partner's content in terms of topic, feeling, depth of feeling, and significance of the circumstance. For example, if your partner had just talked to you about his feelings surrounding the death of a relative, his sense of sadness and loss, and you share your own feelings about the death of your pet cat, it is obvious that you match the topic of death and sadness and loss and perhaps even the depth of feelings; but the significance of the two events, comparing the death of a relative to the death of a pet, is a serious mismatch and could have a serious negative effect on how your partner perceives you and your ability to empathize and understand how he feels.

As mentioned previously, the appropriateness of sharing depends on timing and matching. Exaggerations through negative practice of inappropriate sharing certainly magnify the occurrence of these elements.

With your short-term interviewing partner deliberately introduce each of these kinds of inappropriate sharing.

First, without regard for what your partner is talking about, share something about a recent event you experienced. You might also prolong the description of it with some details, so that you dominate the talking time for a while.

Following this, try to share something that doesn't quite match some aspects of the things that your partner has been talking about. For example, he may have described something that he thought was funny, and you share a similar incident but thought it was quite serious. Or you might mismatch the general significance of what you share with what your partner has told you.

Again, reverse roles so that you experience such inappropriate sharing and can feel the effects of that on your perceptions of your interviewer.

Inappropriate Interpretation

An interpretation by the counselor implies that the counselor has made some observations or developed some understanding about the client's problems that the client would benefit from knowing about. It is new information for the client, but it should be based on things that the client has shared with the counselor. Such a tactic by the counselor requires that his initial observations have led him to developing some hypotheses about the client that relate to the nature and possibly the resolution of the client's problems. Once these hypotheses have been developed by the counselor, he then goes about the task of accepting or rejecting them, based on still further probing, observing, and interacting with his client. The content of these hypotheses can range from dealing with cause and effect relationships between different issues that the client has talked about, to the client's personal needs or latent feelings about an issue, to an understanding of the dynamics of many of his interpersonal relationships. They could involve such things as rationalization, denial, and exploiting his problem by virtue of benefiting from secondary rewards relative to his communication problem. To arrive at such conclusions about the client takes time. If the counselor's hypotheses are confirmed, he must decide whether it would benefit the client to know about these conclusions, and also when the optimum point in time might be for that benefit to be maximized.

If interpretation is premature, that is, if it is engaged in very early in the relationship, one might wonder if the counselor really had enough time to engage in all of the observational activity required, in thinking through his hypotheses, and then in probing for confirmation.

Also, some interpretations may provide very broad sweeps about the person, his development, his style, and his way of thinking, believing, feeling, and interacting with people. They can be very significant and very painful to a client because, in a sense, the counselor may be saying to the client, "This is your life." As a result, the language of the counselor in expressing his interpretation to the client has to be sensitive, nonpunitive, and take into account the pain that may be associated with what the client is hearing for the first time about himself.

Sometimes, an inappropriately worded interpretation generates denial, hostility, defensiveness, and anger in the client. Sometimes it can generate tears, silence, and sadness, even depression.

Even after an appropriate interpretation, you can expect some silence while the client thinks about what he has just heard. You can also expect some emotional reactions. The counselor's paralinguistic and nonverbal behaviors should communicate that he is still there to help the client, not to accuse him or judge him, even with the painful interpretations he has just shared. If such sensitivity is absent on these occasions, then the potential value of the interpretation may be lost.

SUGGESTED PRACTICE PROJECTS

If you have offered an interpretation without going through the several steps just discussed, you run the risk of being premature or inaccurate. Each step is important to the process of interpretation, and omitting any one of them can have a major effect on your accuracy.

Sometimes, you hear something for the first time that you feel you cannot pass by, like someone who obviously is using his communication problem as an excuse for failing to do something. If you want to practice such an action—knowing in advance that it is a departure from the suggested progression of events—then such practice may help you learn this.

Negative practice of each of the steps in the progression of hypothesizing, observing, accepting or rejecting your hypothesis, deciding whether or not to share your conclusion, and finally interpreting it to your partner, can be helpful. Omitting any of these steps may accentuate their value, especially if you are wrong. But there will be times when you may be right on target on all things without going through this step-by-step progression. It is risky from several standpoints. If you're wrong, you risk your relationship with your client. If you're right, you risk being reinforced on a seductive intermittent schedule that is difficult to extinguish.

Defensiveness

Defensiveness from the counselor usually is associated with his being attacked in some fashion by his client. Our experience has been that defensiveness only fuels the fire for the client. It is not an appropriate way to relate to a client because it means that the counselor has lost his focus on the client, and maybe his desire to be helpful to the client. It is a self-focus, and a loss of his subordinate role in the counseling relationship.

When being verbally attacked by the client, whatever the reason, without regard for its validity, the counselor should permit the client to express himself, without interruption. Let him have his say, express his emotions, his anger, his frustration, his blaming you. When the client's emotions have run their course, the counselor has several choices—none of which are to defend himself. He can express his regret over how the client feels about him, but more importantly, he should try to empathize with the conditions and the feelings of the client at that moment. Reflect his feelings, summarize both feelings and content, show him that you want to understand the nature of his feelings toward you, and try to find out what it is that he wants that is not occurring because of you. There may be an opportunity for the counselor to clarify things in a reasoned way for the client, but such clarification should not be the first thing you do, because it could easily be interpreted by the client as counselor defensiveness or a quick denial by the counselor of what the client is complaining about. If done at all, clarification should come later, after the client has completed what he has to say, and after the counselor has tried to communicate his desire to understand, and to resolve whatever is not going right between them.

It is probably the most natural thing in the world for a person to defend what he has been doing when it has been attacked. It is both a natural and quick response, almost like an unconscious trigger that can go off, even when one is alert to the unhelpful consequences of defending oneself.

SUGGESTED PRACTICE PROJECTS

Dealing with your own defensiveness may take some special training, such as desensitization, wherein a training partner or colleague bombards the counselor-in-training with negative, attacking comments, while the counselor continues to keep his focus, shuts down the trigger of defensiveness, and instead engages in nondefensive counseling tactics, even as the bombardment continues. It isn't easy, but such an experience may enable you to weather such a storm under real counseling conditions.

Is Too Seductive and Flirtatious

The bonds of affection that develop between a counselor and a client are considered to be important to the development of trust that develops between the two participants. Strupp (1972) stated that these feelings are so powerful that the client often submits to the therapist's caring and nurturance and the process of self-examination as a consequence of this affectionate bonding. He further states that it is possible that the client changes out of his or her love for the therapist.

Often, the client can misinterpret these feelings of affection for the counselor as a romantic love relationship. They sometimes overtly act on this misinterpretation and inform the counselor of these feelings. The client has been sharing very private and intimate issues, and on occasion the counselor has shared some of his own matching experiences to be helpful to the client. The affection is not a one-way issue. During these moments of sharing, the counselor also has been developing feelings of affection toward his client. Ideally, this is a type of healthy, unqualified, nonromantic caring for the client's well-being that a subordinate helper should experience in his role as someone who is facilitating the other person's self-discovery and self-actualization.

Both participants can become vulnerable to the affection of the other. Sometimes the counselor also mistakes his feelings for something that goes beyond his helping function, and he may overtly express this or show how he feels in many different ways.

It can come out in the form of prolonged eye contact and flirtatious gaze patterns, making personal comments about the client's physical characteristics, sitting too close to the client, inappropriately touching the client, or touching the client too frequently. It can be subtle or very direct. Each of the participants in such a close working relationship, sharing such personal and intimate things about themselves, may feel very close emotionally to each other. Gratitude, affection, caring, closeness, and intimate sharing are very powerful forces that can easily be abused or misused or misunderstood. A therapeutic relationship that changes to a romantic or sexual relationship is a disaster for both parties. The therapy relationship gives way to the interpersonal relationship. The helper–helpee circumstance is destroyed. The focus and roles of each participant are lost. Any immediate gratifications that may be experienced very quickly fade away, and are replaced by feelings that destroy not only the affection and respect the counselor and the client may have felt for each other, but also destroy any therapeutic gains that the client may have experienced, and the counselor's respect for himself.

Obviously, being flirtatious and seductive, even in its earliest stages, carries a potential for total disaster, and through the diligence of the counselor—and perhaps the awareness of the client—should be nipped in the bud as soon as possible.

SUGGESTED PRACTICE PROJECTS

Obviously, negative practice is not an appropriate approach for dealing with this unwanted and undesirable tactic. The counselor, in a true sense of honest self-examination should determine if he is attracted to his "client," that is, the long-term interviewing partner. If the answer is "yes," then there may be some possibility that you may have consciously or unconsciously revealed that attraction in your interviews with that person. However, whatever the answer might be, the counselor should try to determine from the recordings of the interviews if there is any material that could be identified as seductive.

In addition, you should discuss this issue with your short-term interviewing partner, and explain that you want to find out if there has been anything in your behavior or demeanor, verbally or nonverbally, that could be perceived as being seductive.

If the answer is "yes," then you should try to get into the details of what the person perceived. Try to document it so that you can become more aware of it. It might be something as simple as unconsciously touching someone's arm or shoulder too often. Or it might be some type of habitual penetrating eye contact that could easily be misinterpreted as being seductive. Such feedback should help counselors modify these distracting and possibly misunderstood behaviors so that they do not become factors in your counseling relationship.

CONCLUSION

This has been a long list of tactics that would be considered inappropriate in a counseling interview. The operational definitions, and their potentially destructive consequences on the counseling relationship, hopefully will sensitize you to recognize where and when and under what circumstances they might be occurring in your counseling interviews, with a view toward understanding them, and understanding yourself in relation to them. There were also some suggestions as to what you might do about some of them if they persist. Table 11.1 is a list of these holistic, nonfacilitative attributes and some examples of how they might appear in an interview. Your inspection of this table should provide further sensitivity to their occurrence and help in your recognition of them and ultimate prevention of their occurrence. Their occurrence as a holistic feature of your interview should be recorded in Table A.3 in Appendix A.

TABLE 11.1
Non-Facilitative, Holistic Attributes of the Interview

Attributes		*Example*
Inattentive posture	Counselor:	(Nonverbal: sitting in a position that is directed away from client. Looking at your watch or out a window, or tapping your finger on the desk.)
Gaze averted	Counselor:	(Avoiding appropriate eye contact especially while listening or talking.)
Incongruent affect	Counselor:	Laughing while client is crying. Talking very loud while client is talking softly.
Stereotypic minimal encourager	Counselor:	(Saying the same minimal encouragers without variation, repeatedly, such as "uh-huh" or "I see.")
Questioning impedes or affects agenda	Client: Counselor:	"I was teased by a girl today." "Was she pretty?"
Denies/doesn't reflect feelings	Client: Counselor:	"I felt so rejected." "You shouldn't jump so quickly to conclusions."
Lengthy response	Counselor:	(Responses should be brief and to the point.)
Self-focus	Counselor:	"I remember once when I was rejected. I just laughed at her, and told her off. I made her cry, and then I felt guilty and apologized."
Inappropriate topic change	Client: Counselor:	"I apologized too, but I don't know why." "Tell me about that other girl you know."
Reinforces superficial content	Counselor:	"You're right, it is a beautiful day, a great day for swimming."
Shows disrespect	Counselor:	"That's no reason to quit."
Shows discomfort	Client: Counselor:	"You've been talking to my mother." "God, how could you think I would ever do that?"
Judgmental	Counselor:	"How could you say that about her. You know she loves you."

(Continued)

TABLE 11.1
(Continued)

Attributes		*Example*
Gives advice	Counselor:	"I think you should apologize to her right away."
Inappropriate interruption	Counselor:	"Whoa, hold up. You can't sit there and tell me that."
Premature/inappropriate confrontation	Counselor:	"What you're saying now isn't what you told me yesterday."
Inappropriate sharing	Counselor:	"I understand how you feel about your father's death. I felt the same way when my dog died."
Is too personal and seductive	Counselor:	"It's hard to imagine anyone rejecting you. You're so beautiful. You're quite wonderful."
Inappropriate interpretation	Counselor:	"From what you just told me, it seems that your mother and father have some serious problems to work out." (Interpretation should be about the client, not about others that he may be talking about.)
Defensiveness	Client:	"I've been coming here once a week for four weeks and all we do is talk. When are you going to start working on my speech problem? This is costing me a lot of money."
	Counselor:	"I can't work on your speech until I get to know you better. I don't even know what's wrong with your speech yet. It's called a diagnosis. I need to do this so that you can get covered by your insurance."
	Client:	"But four weeks?"
	Counselor:	"I know, but it takes a while to do this accurately and thoroughly."

12

SPECIAL CLIENT POPULATIONS

Up to this point, our considerations of the processes of counseling have dealt almost exclusively with a system that depends on people listening and talking to each other. We have assumed that the participants shared a linguistic system that enabled them to respond to each other, relative to the verbal and nonverbal expressions by each of them, with a special focus on the client and his expressions of feelings and emotions, and the circumstances for those feelings.

An intact linguistic system, which includes both understanding and producing linguistic symbols, as well as a sensorimotor system for receiving and producing speech sounds, has come to be the foundation for the counseling process.

Periodically we have suggested that the counselor should also be "listening with the third ear," as Reik (1949) put it; that is, that the counselor should learn to perceive feelings and emotions that are never put into words—and once perceived, to then put them into some word form to be reflected back to the client. But even in this instance, "words" and "language" are still the basic currency for the process.

There are, however, a significant number of people who have communication problems and cannot talk at all, or only very little. Some also cannot hear, nor understand what they do hear. Some cannot put their feelings into words, even though they may understand what they hear, and know what they want to say. In addition, they may not hear or understand the various types of comments and invitations and reflections that may be offered by the counselor.

These are those individuals whose communication problems are associated with sensorimotor problems of the speech and hearing mechanism, with brain damage, and with severe emotional difficulties and social withdrawal. In such diagnostic categories as deafness, autism, aphasia, cerebral palsy, learning disabled, attention deficit disorder, Alzheimer's disease, Parkinson's, and the mentally retarded, their intellectual systems, memory, ability to abstract, and ability to perceive patterns of events, as well as their receptive and expressive linguistic skills and social competence, may be affected. The occurrence and degree of such disabilities vary from diagnosis to diagnosis and from person to person within each category. But as A. Holland (2002) pointed out relative to aphasia, their emotional systems, in terms of specific brain damage, are still intact and operating. They "feel," and suffer psychological pain. They know frustration, a sense of isolation, and a lowered self-esteem. Such individuals and their families are in need of and could also benefit from counseling.

Wiig and Secord (1998) cited numerous observations of the needs of the learning disabled for counseling. They further pointed out that the process of counseling must take into account the particular and specific communication challenges offered by these individuals. We would extend Wiig and Secord's invitation to all of those clinicians who have the special experience and background for accessing language with these types of communication problems, to bring their expertise to the process of counseling, and to the need for modifying the traditional counseling procedures that are so dependent on relatively intact linguistic and speech systems. For these populations where speech and language may be almost nonexistent, the "Counselor–Speech Clinician" will have to develop other creative and unique methods for dealing with the emotional issues associated with these problems.

We try to suggest some principles and guidelines, and some specific tactics that might be helpful.

All of this assumes that the counselor is approaching this task with a strong background in the nature and dynamics and therapy for the communication problems of his client.

There are at least four major issues to consider that can get us started toward managing this challenge. As we get into these start-up issues, more issues will probably evolve.

1. The counselor must determine as accurately as possible the client's needs and goals, in terms of speech and language as well as counseling.
2. The counselor must access the client's residual language and his expressions of emotions and feelings as well as the content and context of the social situations and circumstances related to those feelings.
3. The counselor must try to increase the understandability of what he is saying to the client.

4. If some means other than oral speech are to be used, the counselor should try to keep to a minimum the time intervals between his comments and the client's response. This caution is specifically in connection with the counselor's or the client's use of devices, pictures, reading or writing of responses, and so on, during the interview. Try to make it appear as "conversational" as possible even though oral speech may be augmented by other means.

NEEDS AND GOALS

Kagan, Winckel, and Shumway (1996), in their film *Supported Conversation for Aphasic Adults—Enhancing Conversation Access* discussed the emotional needs of the client and offered a model for accessing language.

As they so aptly stated, the aphasic needs a companion, someone who will provide support for their efforts. They need warmth and acceptance and patience; someone who can say "I know that you know" to the aphasic, and mean it.

A. Holland (2002) pointed out that although there may have been severe damage to the brain, that portion of the brain that focuses on emotion is usually still operating, enabling the client to feel the same feelings that all of us feel. Given the seriousness of their physical and neurological and communication problems, it is not too difficult to empathize, to sense what must be going on inside the person, even though he may not be able to put it into words. His sense of loss of what he used to be able to do, his frustration and helplessness that he can't move some portion of his body, or say what he wants to say, or that he feels left out of conversation, and can't demonstrate his social or linguistic competence, are each very significant factors in his daily condition and functioning. Perhaps more than in any of the examples earlier in the book, your role as both a speech pathologist and a counselor become closely integrated. There is no vacillating, no role changing for the client from person centered (client centered) to counselor directed. The interaction is primarily counselor directed and counselor initiated. In some ways, your communication with such patients is like a role play for you, wherein you empathize from your own experiences and from the experiences you have had with other clients what the client might be thinking or feeling at any given moment, and this then becomes the content of what is introduced and being considered.

ACCESSING CONTENT AND FEELINGS

The principle for helping the client to communicate his feelings and the content of the situations related to those feelings is to keep his mode of responding as simple and short as possible. In many instances, this means doing just the opposite of those things you were practicing and learning and integrating into your interviews in the earlier portions of the book.

Keep remembering that the emotional system is still operating even though the language system is not.

Generally, the counselor should word his responses so that they are closed, requiring little or no composition by the client. One-word answers, "yes" and "no" affirmations or denials of statements composed by the counselor, are the primary vehicle. The responses by the client may include something as simple as head nodding and smiling, indicating agreement or disagreement with what the counselor has just said to him. This puts a very heavy load on the counselor for composing material that is pertinent to the issues that are significant for the client. Earlier, several times, we mentioned empathizing; getting into the client's shoes and walking around in his world. This means that you are making educated guesses about things, and that the client can either accept and affirm or deny and reject, either with a word or with a gesture.

Sometimes during the interview the client may show you nonverbally through gestures of his head and hands, or total body movement, that he is emoting. He may cry, shout, repeatedly produce a perseverative chain of nonsense syllables that sounds like gibberish. These may be important and significant emotional expressions, and should not be cut off or terminated by the clinician. The client may need these emotional ventilations and expressions, and should be permitted to show them and be comfortable enough with you to feel that you accept and understand what he is doing. In fact, Kagan et al. (1996) strongly suggested that you say to him, "I know, I understand what you're going through."

In addition to any words you use, you might also use devices that caption what would usually be your oral speech as an auditory stimulus that he might not understand, into a voice-activated visual stimulus that he can read. This might be especially useful in counseling the deaf, as well as with certain types of aphasia.

Sometimes your verbalizing should be supported with pictures, or multiple-choice questions or multiple-choice pictures, as a way of enhancing your interaction.

Kagan et al. (1996) emphasized that you should try to think of these various methods of accessing residual language as ramps to his language, like the ramps that are used for the physically handicapped to enable physical access.

You have to try to access his sense of isolation, his anger, his depression and sadness, his embarrassment, his loss and his frustration, and give him every chance to demonstrate his linguistic and social competence.

Being physically close, with good eye contact, and occasionally touching the client, are also ways of communicating your caring, your affection and concern, and your availability.

In addition, you may find that having the client write his response may be a way of accessing his talking. Writing by the counselor may also be helpful in combination with the counselor's talking as a way of enhancing the client's understanding of what you are communicating. Using concrete objects or watching real events may also help.

Again, try to keep the time interval short between your composition with whatever augmentative devices you may employ and your client's response, with whatever augmentative devices he may use.

If you're dealing with the past, and past feelings, it might not be so critical to keep the time intervals brief. But a long time interval between experiencing a current feeling and somehow reporting it may distort the experience.

In Table 12.1, a few examples of inappropriate and appropriate tactics might be helpful.

These are just a few examples of what might be helpful and what might not be helpful in your interactions with your client. Counseling with people who have limited linguistic, memory, and reasoning skills taps into

TABLE 12.1
Inappropriate and Appropriate Tactics

Inappropriate Counselor Tactics	*Appropriate Counselor Tactics*
1. "Hi, Mr. Doe. Tell me why you came to see me today."	"I know you have some problems. I'm here to help." (open instruction)
2. "You're having some problems, right? Is it pain? No. Are you sad? Yes, I know it's hard on you."	"What kind of problems are they?" (open question)
3. Silent listening	"Do you understand me when I talk?" (open invitation) "Yes, good."
4. "I can't understand what you just said." (open invitation)	"Do you know the words but you just can't say them? Yes! Let me write out what I think you want to say. If I'm right just nod your head."
5. Silence (open invitation)	"Can you write out what you want to say?"
6. "After she told you about your illness, what did you feel?" (open question) "I think I would have cried." (Counselor composes what he thinks the feeling was, reflects it to the client, and shares his own emotional reaction to the situation.)	"You must have felt very frightened."
7. "If you can't talk it's going to be a tough go." (pessimistic evaluation)	"Do you want to try the typing device to tell me about it? Fine, go ahead."
8. "If you don't know what you want to accomplish here, then I'm not sure where to start." (not accepting of client)	"I know you know. And it's my job and my goal to help you to show me what you mean. Stick with me. We'll get it eventually."

your most creative talents. For such people, you should try to get a picture of their daily routine, where they go, how they generally communicate their needs to their caretakers, the nature of their residual language, who they communicate with and how they communicate with them, what they do, how they spend their time and where they spend their time, what they would enjoy doing, and how they feel about all of these things. The client's involvement with family and community as well as with health issues may well be the focus of your efforts from a situational standpoint. The dramatic changes in his routines—occupationally, socially, and in personal caretaking—are also themes for counseling these patients. The client needs to be helped to recognize and accept both his weaknesses and his strengths, and to develop a realistic yet positive attitude and approach to his life as it now is. Clinging to the past, and focusing on what used to be, generates a wide array of feelings, including his sadness, his denial, his lack of accepting the reality of his current status, and often anger and depression. Each of these may become your content categories for exploring the feelings associated with these situational issues.

Accessing the client's residual language, especially in the emotional sphere, will require a great deal of empathizing and composing by you. It is likely to be the most exhausting and creative endeavor you will ever undertake.

In addition to the patient who cannot talk, there is a need to deal with the patient's caretakers—spouse, family, and close significant others. Their attitudes, feelings, beliefs, and actions can have a direct bearing on how the patient functions. Because of their role as helpers, they need to be brought into the total rehabilitation process. They need information, and a reality-based approach to the patient. In order to accomplish this, it is usually necessary to work through and explore the feelings of the family through counseling as well. Their self-pity, grief, feelings of being overwhelmed, and possibly resentment and anger, may have to be dealt with before they can ever become helpful to the patient. They often feel much like the patient himself—that they are quite alone. For this reason, counseling for both the patient and his family may be enhanced if the patients are seen in small groups. This is also true for the families and caretakers of these patients. Knowing that there are others facing the same issues, the sharing of incidents and feelings among them, and sometimes the sharing of resolutions to these issues among the participants can only be experienced in a group arrangement.

Boles and Lewis (1998) offered a less common approach to counseling for the problem of aphasia, by applying the concepts of "Solution Focused Couples Therapy." They have been very generous in their sharing of transcripts and their qualitative analyses of this type of counseling for aphasics and their spouses for use in this manual. The following material, with their permission, has been extracted from one actual Solution Focused Couples Therapy session from a series of 14 sessions, that an aphasiologist (Boles), and a social worker (Lewis) conducted with an aphasic woman and her spouse. As they pointed out, "Because many patients are either married or have an interpersonal relationship with a significant other, it is not unusual for an aphasiologist to recommend couples therapy." Solution Focused Therapy (SFT) has proven to be successful in marital counseling, for mixed marriages, as well as for individuals with aphasia.

According to Boles and Lewis (1998) the principles of SFT are: (a) determine what the client wants, (b) look for what is working and do more of that, and (c) identify what is not working and do something different. Exceptions to problems are emphasized rather than pursuing the "cause."

The qualitative analysis involved the identification of exemplars from the transcript of the therapy session that demonstrate the specific tactics being employed interchangeably by the two cotherapists and the nature of the interactions among the four participants.

Of necessity, to enable the reader to understand the dynamics of these tactics, a series of successive responses from the participants are quoted, followed by a brief comment about the strategy being employed.

In this particular study, the client is referred to as Lydia. She had a left middle cerebral artery infarct some 10 years ago. She is aged 51 and has been diagnosed as having a mild anomic aphasia. Her speech and language are occasionally lengthy but often agrammatic. Her husband, who is referred to as Frank, is aged 61, nonaphasic, and retired. He has received individual therapy for depression. Frank had reported some difficulties in their relationship that led to the recommendation for couples therapy.

Numerous issues were discussed during this session, including (a) affection shown by Frank toward Lydia, (b) Lydia's distracting Frank while he drives, (c) Frank's depression, and (d) Lydia feeling like a "loser."

While discussing these topics, each of the four participants used certain conversational techniques and patterns in their interaction (i.e., exemplars). After a brief period of small talk, termed a "neutral zone," ML (Lewis) opened the session.

ML's conversational patterns included (a) opening the session, (b) finding exceptions and emphasizing the positive, and (c) giving assignments and pursuing the assignment across turns.

Exemplar 1

3. LB (Boles): is it too hot?
4. ML: no

5. LB: (laughs) I've never heard her say it's too hot.
6. ML: never too hot.
7. ML: so how are you?

In (7), ML directed the participants away from the neutral zone (3–6) and into an opening—similar to check in on their status. In (10–12), Frank's comments moved them back into the neutral zone, but ML persisted with the opening.

Exemplar 3

40. Lydia: been to Mexico? (referring to an earlier comment by Frank about her Mexican earrings)
41. ML: Mhmm yeah.
42. ML: so you said you were doing good. Right? Better now?

In (42) is another attempt by ML to execute an opening.

Finding Exceptions/Emphasizing the Positive

As mentioned earlier, exceptions are emphasized in SFT. ML uses this technique several times, as follows in a discussion about getting taxes filed by the April 15 deadline.

Exemplar 5

53. Frank: I have to make a special trip sometime.
54. ML: But I'm impressed that you are going to get them in the mail today.
55. Frank: Yeah it feels pretty good.

Later in the session the participants discussed Frank's showing of affection toward Lydia. Twice in the previous week he had given her "back scratches," an unusual display of affection for him.

Exemplar 6

146. Frank: It's not very prolonged but I love to see her happy.
147. Frank: And I realize I'm . . . I'm hard to live with almost all the time.
148. Frank: So I like to break out of it.

149. ML: I'm curious about how you decided to give her back scratches.
150. ML: What was it?

It wasn't clear whether Frank would emphasize the positive (146, 148) or the negative (147). ML again emphasized the positive (149–150). In fact, ML made no secret of her strategy:

Exemplar 7

153. ML: You know what I'd like to do is I'd like to analyze the strengths.
154. ML: Instead of analyze the problems.
155. ML: So here's a strength.
156. ML: You went and gave her a back rub.

The Assignment. ML regularly gave Frank and Lydia "assignments," a habit that Lydia welcomed and Frank resisted. In the following segment, ML proposed such an assignment. Frank had just expressed displeasure and occasional anger because Lydia had a habit of combing his hair in the car while he was driving.

Exemplar 8

315. ML: Okay would that be something you could agree to do is not to comb his hair?
316. ML: In the car?
317. ML: Comb or brush.
318. Lydia: Yes.

The giving of an assignment was considered an important aspect of therapy to ML. It was felt that an increased investment in the therapy process was achieved with these assignments. ML later returned to "the assignment."

Exemplar 9

403. ML: But I guess what I hear is that this really bothers Frank.
404. ML: And I wonder if you're willing to stop doing it in the car at least.
405. Lydia: Oh, in the car, yeah.

ML's strategy of repeating the assignment may have been motivated by Lydia's communication impairment, or simply by her desire to solidify the agreement.

The next portion of the exemplars deals with LB's exemplars. LB's conversational patterns included (a) finding exceptions and emphasizing the positive, (b) conversation trouble repairs, (c) affirming the two clients, and (d) using humor.

Finding Exceptions/Emphasizing the Positive by LB with regard to Frank's scratching Lydia's back follows in exemplars 12 to 15.

Exemplar 12

141. LB: How was that during those moments?
142. Frank: I like to I tried to uh tried to be more aware of, uh, thinking of Lydia.
143. Frank: And then feeling, that is, in terms of my busy-ness with other things.
144. LB: So during those moments, are you able to let go of those other things?

A few minutes later LB asked Frank to elaborate further on this display of affection.

Exemplar 13

190. LB: Is it more of a tuning out?
191. LB: I mean, what is, what is that?
192. Frank: I think it's getting more in touch with the deepest feelings I have.
193. Frank: They're almost always covered up.

The conversation turned to the "silent treatment" about halfway into the session. Frank and Lydia agreed that Frank had been giving her the silent treatment less frequently. Lydia recalled only two silent treatments since the previous session, 10 days earlier. LB asked for elaboration.

Exemplar 14

545. LB: Frank I want to ask you about that.
546. LB: Because to emphasize the good things that are happening it seems like you have an increased awareness of how hurtful they might be.

547. LB: How did that happen?
548. LB: Just trying to think of other things.

Moments later LB said the following to Frank:

Exemplar 15

575. LB: . . . helping her realize an improved quality of life.
576. LB: You seem—your affect even seems more up.
577. LB: And I just wonder if you're experiencing it that way or . . .
578. Frank: It is right now.

Conversation Repair. It seems inevitable in a session that includes an individual with aphasia that conversation repair (Boles, 1997) would occur. In the following segment, Lydia talked about the back scratches.

Exemplar 16

98. Lydia: Now sitting on the sofa. . . .
99. Lydia: . . . but in the kitchen and everywhere it's good.
100. LB: When you said sitting on the sofa, is that where he does the back rub?
101. LB: On the, on the sofa.
102. LB: Is that what you mean?

In the following segment LB and ML unsuccessfully attempted to repair a conversation segment. Lydia finally accomplished the task herself.

488. LB: Oh so in the car it matters whether there's grouchiness or not?
489. ML: No, no what I get (understand) is in the car you do it no matter what (be)cause he's a captive.
490. ML: He's your—he can't move away from you.
491. ML: Is that right?
492. Lydia: No, no, no.
493. Lydia: In the morning he's grouchy.
494. Lydia: Comb your hair.
495. Lydia: No, not now.
496. ML: Okay.
497. LB: Oh, okay.

498. Lydia: So out the door, ehh. (noise indicating his hair looks horrible)
499. LB: So you didn't get your chance in the house?
500. LB: 'Cause he was grouchy?
501. Lydia: Yeah.

Affirmations. Therapists, whether aphasiologists or couples therapists, have a tendency to affirm their clients. The following segment illustrates LB's response to Frank after he has talked about his motivation for being kind to Lydia.

Exemplar 19

221. Frank: Well I think predominantly it's trying to tell her how important she is to me.
222. Frank: It's kind of a feeble way of doing it I guess.
223. LB: Really?
224. LB: It doesn't sound feeble to me.
225. Frank: The meaning is clear but I can't stop (unintelligible word).
226. LB: You know Lydia has expressed how important touch is to her.
227. LB: And so, I mean, I would urge you not to downplay how important it is.

Humor. It has been the experience of the authors (Boles and Lewis) that carefully placed humor can be a useful tool in the therapeutic arsenal. Humor is a pattern used often by LB.

Exemplar 20

394. Lydia: Dances and pirouettes and keep it's half still and comb your hair. (laughs)
395. LB: Oh you mean he tries to avoid you combing it?
396. Lydia: Yeah.
397. LB: (laughs) So you're (to Frank) getting good.
398. LB: You're aiming with this comb at this moving target.
399. Lydia: Yeah. (laughs)
400. Frank: She's getting good too.
401. LB: So you really have to learn some more moves to this dance then?

The exemplars or conversational patterns considered thus far have focused on the two therapists, and their strategies for conducting the Solution Focused Couples therapy with this couple. However, it is also important to become sensitive and aware of the patterns of the clients, so that you might recognize when they need your help.

Boles and Lewis have also conducted a detailed analysis of each of the clients in this session. Space limits how much detail we can provide about these exemplars, but fortunately the authors have summarized the information and we can provide enough to sensitize you and perhaps encourage you to read their publication in *Aphasiology*. Therefore we briefly highlight this information with minimal reference to the transcript.

Lydia's patterns included (a) fading out and other intonational strategies as a way of asking for conversational help, (b) qualifying her statements, and (c) reenacting a scene to illustrate a point. The authors pointed out that most of the time her intonation actually guided her listeners toward her intent.

Frank's patterns included (a) preoccupation with tasks, (b) qualifying positive statements with negative ones and vice versa, (c) responses related to feelings, and (d) affirming Lydia.

There are two exemplars related to Frank's expression of feelings that are quite moving, and would be valuable to become aware of as a somewhat common experience in this type of therapy. The authors pointed out that "It is perhaps common during couples therapy for the expression of feelings to arise." It was interesting to note Frank's responses when feelings were discussed. Just prior to one of the segments of conversation, Frank had stated he had "deep feelings" that enabled him to give back scratches to Lydia. LB pushed further with his inquiry into the feelings a few moments later.

Exemplar 29

218. LB: Well if you don't mind I want to go to those feelings that you go toward.
219. LB: So that some kind of feelings drive you towards Lydia's back.
220. Frank: Mhmm.
221. LB: What are those feelings?
222. Frank: Well I think it's just trying to just tell her how important she is to me.

Although LB did not pursue this topic further, "importance" was not the deep feeling LB had expected.

Late in the session, ML asked Frank and Lydia to face one another. The following segment occurred while they were in that position.

Exemplar 30

958. ML: Can you tell Lydia how you feel about her?
959. Frank: (to ML) The love?
960. ML: Mhmm.
961. Frank: Yeah—infinite caring about you Lydia.
962. ML: So "I infinitely care about you."
963. Frank: Yeah, and I want you to have just the best possible quality of life.
964. ML: Can you tell her that again?
965. Frank: Lydia I feel totally devoted to you.
966. Frank: Total love.
967. Lydia: Really.
968. Frank: Of course.

Frank's question (959) and Lydia's surprise (967) were perhaps indicative of Frank's awkwardness when stating his feelings. Even after ML confirmed the purpose of facing one another (960), it took Frank three more turns to say "total love."

The authors pointed out that many of the tactics employed in this particular application of Solution Focused Couples Therapy might be just as appropriate in individual counseling, and also that the cotherapists, in this case a social worker and a speech pathologist, could easily move in and out of each other's roles and perspectives with appropriate training. It again demonstrates the multidimensionality of communication problems, as well as the multidimensionality of the helpers.

It would be interesting to explore how this particular approach to conversational repair, and clarification, might be combined with the techniques discussed earlier in this chapter, involving the tactics offered by A. Holland (2002) regarding (a) keeping responses simple—"yes/no" answers, by having the therapist compose the verbal response requiring a simple affirmation or denial; (b) using AAC devices to enhance and access residual language; and (c) encouraging emotional responses, both verbal and nonverbal, and using the tactics of Kagan et al. (1996) regarding multiple choice, reading and writing, and/or captioning techniques to enhance communication, especially with more severely handicapped aphasics.

Many of these people have irreversible medical problems and irreversible communication problems. If you can succeed, even in limited ways, to help them live their lives more positively, you will know a sense of contributing, and a sense of accomplishment that will become an indelible part of you. You will also experience a bonding with that client and his family that will never disappear.

13

SOME COMMENTS ABOUT THE OUTCOMES OF THERAPY

Can a speech problem be cured? The answer to this question relates directly to how much we know about its cause. A cure denotes that the causes have been eliminated, or are no longer operative, and that therefore the problem is permanently and forever gone from a person's life.

The cause or causes of a multidimensional problem like a communication problem may include behavioral, cognitive, affective, physiological, and societal factors. This suggests that a single cause for this type of problem may never be identified. As a result, there is always a possibility that even after the most successful experiences in therapy, under certain circumstances the pretherapy feelings, beliefs, attitudes, and even speech behavior may return for varying amounts of time. What therapy has done is perhaps reduce the probability of the occurrence of behaviors and attitudes associated with a particular communication problem under certain adverse emotional, physical, and social circumstances. Therapy has also increased the probability of the occurrence of appropriate speech and attitudinal reactions under adverse conditions, because of what was learned in therapy.

As you gain experience as a clinician, you soon come to realize that your clients are under your influence, but not under your control. Decisions about goals for a particular client are negotiated with the client, and may vary from person to person. These goals, in turn, influence the overall strategies, clinical tactics, and criteria for terminating therapy. All of these issues therefore become a shared responsibility between you and the person with whom you are working.

There are at least five classes of variables that affect success of therapy, though success may be defined differently from problem to problem, from therapy to therapy, and from person to person.

One of these variables is the client, with his history of the problem, his motivation, his personality attributes, his readiness for change, and his prior history of therapy.

A second variable is the amount of support available from the client's family or people who are important to him, as he tries to conquer his problems.

A third variable is the amount of stress the client lives with day in and day out. Some of this stress may not be related to his speaking, although some of it may. If too much stress overloads the system in the same time frame, it can overwhelm the client in his attempt to change his speech.

A fourth variable is the particular system of therapy being employed, its validity and comprehensiveness, and whether it addresses the totality of the problem, and is understood by the client.

Finally, there is you, the caring, knowledgeable, available clinician. It is your style and wisdom and technical knowledge that bring therapy to life.

Some of these variables are more under your control than others, for example, those that relate to your own behavior and attitudes as a clinician, and to your decisions about a system of therapy.

However, you may be able to influence the client's motivation and readiness to change, and even his perceptions of past failures in therapy. You may be able to mobilize or inspire his family and other significant persons in his life to be helpful. You may even help the client to resolve certain stressful issues in his life.

This is the area where the tactics of counseling come into significance. In the context of therapy for a communication problem, you will quickly become aware of your "in and out" role: switching between counseling activity and speech therapy. At times, these counseling tactics will be surrounded by speech therapy activities. At other times these counseling tactics will be periodically punctuated by a speech therapy activity, whereas at yet other times the counseling tactics will be embedded within speech therapy activities. They can be executed separately, or come together and operate in some kind of tandem or combined fashion. Your judgment about how and when you integrate counseling and speech therapy could be an important factor in the eventual outcome of therapy.

The following is a transcript of a segment of a counseling interview that demonstrates the constant switching of roles by a speech clinician. He moves back and forth from using client-centered counseling tactics to using very directive instructional tactics that are more associated with speech therapy. For the most part, the content of the issues is concerned with strategies for dealing with Fred's speech problem. However, they also address in general his willingness to take risks, his relationship with his wife, and his work. The analysis focuses on the clinician's behavior, indicating when he is behaving more like a speech therapist and when he is engaging in tactics associated with counseling. Note how he moves in and out of these various functions of counseling and speech therapy—although the target is for the most part the client's speech.

Fred has a problem with stuttering. He received 2 weeks of intensive therapy for his problem 2 years before this interview. He kept in touch with his therapist for about 6 months, during which he progressed through the final stages of his therapy. It was mutually decided that regular contact was no longer necessary. Except for an occasional telephone call or holiday card there has been no contact with the therapist. After about a year and a half of no contact, he arranged for this appointment. Only a small portion of that follow-up interview is provided to demonstrate the dual functioning of counseling and speech therapy during this session.

TRANSCRIPT OF COUNSELING SESSION

1. Fred: Hi, Dr. S., it's good to see you.
2. Dr. S.: Hi Fred, yeah, it's been a while.
3. Dr. S.: How're things going for you? (open invitation to talk)
4. Fred: Some good. Some not so good.
5. Dr. S.: How do you mean? (open question)
6. Fred: Well, with my wife, they're going a lot better.
7. Dr. S.: A lot better? (echoing—verbal following and attending)
8. Fred: Yeah, she understands now, how I have to do things for myself instead of the way I used to let her do things.
9. Dr. S.: Was there trouble with that for her or for you? (closed question)
10. Fred: I was tempted to let it go on, but I knew better.
11. Dr. S.: What happened? (open question)
12. Fred: She thought I didn't need her anymore, and then she jumped to some crazy idea that I didn't love her anymore.
13. Dr. S.: So then . . . (incomplete phrase—minimal encourager)
14. Fred: It was easy to show her that I still needed her but in different ways and showing her I loved her—that was easy.
15. Dr. S.: The bad part of what's been happening? (open question)

16. Fred: It's my speech. Well not really my speech, it's this feeling I get, some tension in my stomach and throat.
17. Dr. S.: When does this happen? (open question)
18. Fred: I can't really predict it. Almost anytime. But I get a little advance warning. Sometimes when I'm on the phone.
19. Dr. S.: What do you do when you feel that tension? (open question)
20. Fred: I stop and try to relax.
21. Dr. S.: Does that help? (closed question)
22. Fred: No.
23. Dr. S.: Do you remember anything that you did back when you were in therapy? (closed question)
24. Fred: What do you mean?
25. Dr. S.: About running your words together. (giving information, teaching)
26. Fred: Oh yeah, I remember.
27. Dr. S.: Fred, say these sounds after I do. ahahah . . . eeeee. (Fred says the sounds)
28. Dr. S.: Now, tell me your name and address, running the words together. How does that feel? (teaching)
29. Fred: Good. Easy, relaxed.
30. Dr. S.: Any tension in your throat or stomach? (closed question)
31. Fred: Nope. None.
32. Dr. S.: Now, where do you go from here with that feeling? (open question)
33. Fred: I guess I need to practice it a little.
34. Dr. S.: Maybe a lot. (giving guidance—functioning as a speech therapist)
35. Dr. S.: Maybe even some specific contracts. (giving guidance—functioning as a speech therapist)
36. Fred: You mean like with my wife?
37. Dr. S.: Would that help? (closed question)
38. Fred: A little. I need to practice it in harder places.
39. Dr. S.: How are things going at work? (open question)
40. Fred: That's where the problem is. I'm supposed to get a promotion next month. Oh, yes, I told them about my work with you too.
41. Dr. S.: How'd it feel, doing that? (open question)
42. Fred: I was nervous about doing it, but I felt great afterward.

43. Fred: But the promotion. I know it's a good thing. But I'm afraid.

44. Dr. S.: You're afraid of your promotion. (paraphrasing content and reflecting feeling)

45. Fred: It's my speech. I'm going to have to do a lot more talking, and under pressure.

46. Dr. S.: Where does it stand now? (open question)

47. Fred: I accepted it, but I'm scared I'm going to screw up.

48. Dr. S.: Screw up . . . (verbal following, echoing, minimal encourager)

49. Fred: Yeah, you know, my speech.

50. Dr. S.: What do you feel you want to do? Here's a chance to get ahead, but it's risky for you. I understand what you're feeling, both the joy and the fear. (reflecting feeling and confronting him with his conflict)

51. Dr. S.: Do you remember back when you were in therapy? Does any of this sound familiar? (closed question)

52. Fred: You mean about taking risks. Yeah.

53. Dr. S.: Yes, about taking risks, but more than that . . . about using your speech problem as a way to avoid things. It was your excuse for possible failures. (paraphrasing content and giving an interpretation)

54. Fred: Yeah, I remember. You told me that using my speech as an excuse was holding me back. But I'm afraid, really afraid of what might happen with my job.

55. Dr. S.: Have you talked to your wife about any of this? (closed question and change of topic)

56. Fred: Yeah, now that I've become so proactive about practicing my new speech she thinks I'm a damn hero.

57. Dr. S.: A hero? Why a hero? (echoing and open question)

58. Fred: Because of what I'm doing. You know. Doing things I'm afraid of. But I don't want to be a hero. I'm still afraid. I'm afraid of things that everyone else takes for granted.

59. Dr. S.: Where'd you get the idea that you were going to lead a life that had no fear in it? Everyone has fears. And with what you lived with all your life, it wouldn't be normal if you weren't afraid. (confrontation in the form of a question and clarification)

60. Dr. S.: Do you remember what happened when you did those things you were afraid of, that carried risks with it? (closed question that is to function like an open question)

61. Fred: Yeah, after a while, I wasn't so afraid of them anymore.
62. Dr. S.: Think Fred: How could that apply to what's going on right now with how you feel about your job? (open question)
63. Fred: I see where you're going. You want me to do some talking contracts at work. (self-discovery by Fred)
64. Dr. S.: How would you organize that? (open question)
65. Fred: Well, if I could figure out what some of those new talking situations were going to be like, and actually practice talking in them, even before my promotion starts. I see . . . I'd be way ahead of the game. Maybe even some of those things I'm afraid of . . . I could practice monitoring my speech and get control and the fear might go away, I mean get used to those things even before I have to face them. (self-discovery leading to action by Fred)
66. Dr. S.: Fred, do you realize what you've just done? (closed question designed to function as an open question)
67. Fred: (Fred smiled) I think so. I think I just fired you.
68. Dr. S.: You solved it Fred. You solved it without me. This is as good as it gets, Fred. (Dr. S. and Fred were both laughing)

The counseling session continued, and led into a long discussion of Fred's past risk taking, his fears, and his views about his future, with Fred eagerly taking the lead about each of these issues.

In reviewing the transcribed segment of this therapy session, you can see that many counseling techniques and tactics were embedded in material that addressed his speech and his speech problem. In these instances, the client-centered approach was utilized for dealing with his speech, except in numbers 23, 25, 27, 28, 30, 34, and 35 where Dr. S. was functioning less as a counselor and more as a speech therapist who was teaching his client what to do about his speech.

In the portion about his promotion at work, Dr. S. was functioning primarily as a client-centered counselor, trying to get Fred to discover for himself what he could be doing about his problem. When Fred developed his own ideas and strategies about his therapy, Dr. S. was quite reinforcing and supportive of what he had done.

This transcript of a speech therapy session shows that there are times and opportunities to approach the focus on changing speech (i.e., functioning as a speech clinician and engaging in speech therapy) while embedding that focus within the tactics of client-centered counseling.

At these times, the client is urged to problem solve, and to figure out for himself what his strategies might be for dealing with his speech—in or out of the therapy session—to discern strategies that might be helpful in changing or maintaining a particular speech pattern.

The clinician should be on the alert for such opportunities, because self-insights and self-designed strategies may be more durable (if appropriate) and acceptable than those offered by the clinician.

However, all of the issues and variables that affect the outcome of therapy, including the emotional issues that are addressed through counseling, are open to many influences in addition to your own. They are under the control of people and circumstances well outside your sphere of functioning.

When all of these classes of variables coalesce and come together in the right way, the chances are that the outcome of therapy will be good. But if even one of them is out of sync, then a positive outcome can be jeopardized.

You can only do what you can do. You must recognize not only your own limitations, but the value of your client (with your support) taking on the responsibility for being active in resolving these other issues in his life that are under his control and not yours. You can show him the way and the routes, but he must take the time to smell the roses.

SUMMARY AND CONCLUSIONS

Throughout this book, we have emphasized the relationship between you and your client. It is this relationship that makes the immediate effects of the conditioning tactics for changing speech durable. The process of therapy, a process of change in and of itself, can be stressful, and can constitute problems. The client has a temporary but deep need of you for this period of his life, and there is a special human quality required for this special therapeutic experience.

In our view, the application of behavior modification principles to therapy does not negate the need and value of counseling. They go hand in hand, and complement each other. We do not rush helter-skelter through our sessions, piling up high frequencies of target responses. Instead, we may have to move slowly while the client becomes comfortable and adapts to what is happening. We may have to deal with the client's feelings as he develops new beliefs and understandings and expectations about himself. These sometimes slow, sometimes exciting, verbal meanderings in the client's cognitive and emotional worlds may be the verbal priming for action by the client. As he develops new speech skills and new hopes for himself, he is also developing an abiding trust in our genuine concern for his well-being.

When we accept the client's faith in us, we also accept the responsibility for helping him to integrate his new behaviors and beliefs into his life, until he no longer needs us.

Your reading and practicing of the materials in this manual has brought you to a completion, but not to a conclusion. You have completed your first, early steps in learning the processes of counseling.

Through your diligence, your self-discipline, your persistence, your commitment, and your honesty about yourself, you have opened a door that gives you an additional perspective about your work with the communicatively disabled. If you walk through that door, you will be entering what I have referred to several times in this manual as "the poetry of the mind."

The human mind, with its many parameters of thought, reasoning, beliefs, and feelings, operates and controls a complicated and dynamic system that allows the human spirit to exist. The more involved you get with any aspect of that system, the more awesome it becomes for the beholder. It is much like a poem with its unique story, and tempo, and emotions and beauty. Your concerns about the sensorimotor aspects, the cognitive aspects, and the behavioral aspects of communication problems are now joined by the emotional aspects of these conditions.

What you have now done once has to be done again and again, until it becomes a natural part of your professional activity.

While thinking about some of the things that go on behind the closed doors of the therapy room, we are reminded of the wistful words of St.-Exupery:

> It is only with the heart that you can see rightly . . .
> What is essential is invisible to the eye . . .
> You become responsible for what you have tamed.
>
> —Antoine de St.-Exupery
> *The Little Prince*, 1943

APPENDIX A

Forms for Evaluating Clinical Interview ______________

Name ______________________________

Observation# ______________ Date______________

TABLE A.1
Specific Facilitative Interviewing Behaviors

	No. Occurrences	*% of Occurrences*	*Total Responses*
A. Verbal following	______	______	______
B. Minimal encouragers to talk	______	______	______
C. Closed questions	______	______	______
D. Open questions	______	______	______
E. Paraphrasing content	______	______	______
F. Reflecting feelings	______	______	______
G. Summarizing content	______	______	______
H. Summarizing feelings	______	______	______
I. Sharing	______	______	______
J. Confrontation	______	______	______
K. Interpretation	______	______	______
L. Clarification	______	______	______
M. Embedded clarification	______	______	______
Total	______		

TABLE A.2
Holistic, Nonspecific, Facilitative Attributes

	Very Poor	*Below Average*	*Average*	*Above Average*	*Outstanding*
A. Client centered	0	1	2	3	4
B. Accepting	0	1	2	3	4
C. Fluent	0	1	2	3	4
D. Concerned/empathic	0	1	2	3	4
E. Relaxed/calm	0	1	2	3	4
F. Doesn't interfere or impede	0	1	2	3	4
G. Does not judge	0	1	2	3	4
H. Does not suggest or give answers	0	1	2	3	4
I. Does not deny feelings	0	1	2	3	4
J. Absence of self-focus	0	1	2	3	4
K. No noticeable disinterest	0	1	2	3	4
L. Tolerates silence	0	1	2	3	4
M. Avoids superficial content	0	1	2	3	4
N. Appropriate topic change	0	1	2	3	4
O. Listens and attends	0	1	2	3	4
P. Appropriate reinforcing	0	1	2	3	4
Q. Generates warmth/trust	0	1	2	3	4
R. Tolerates crying	0	1	2	3	4
S. Accepts emotional language	0	1	2	3	4

TABLE A.3
Holistic, Nonspecific, Nonfacilitative Attributes

A. Inattentive posture	0	1	2	3	4
B. Gaze averted	0	1	2	3	4
C. Incongruent affect	0	1	2	3	4
D. Stereotypic minimal encouragers	0	1	2	3	4
E. Questioning impedes/affects agenda	0	1	2	3	4
F. Denies/doesn't reflect feelings	0	1	2	3	4
G. Lengthy responses	0	1	2	3	4
H. Self-focus	0	1	2	3	4
I. Inappropriate topic change	0	1	2	3	4
J. Reinforces superficial content	0	1	2	3	4
K. Shows disrespect/discomfort/judgmental, and gives advice	0	1	2	3	4
L. Premature/inappropriate confrontation	0	1	2	3	4
M. Inappropriate sharing	0	1	2	3	4
N. Inappropriate interruption	0	1	2	3	4
O. Is too personal/seductive	0	1	2	3	4

Note. A rating of 4 denotes outstanding. For nonfacilitative behaviors it means that the attribute is generally absent, and is viewed as a positive characteristic of the interview. All ratings of (1) for all of the scales is in the nonhelpful direction. All ratings of (4) are in the helpful category.

APPENDIX B

WORDS TO DESCRIBE FEELINGS

Abandoned
Adamant
Adequate
Affectionate
Afraid
Aggravated
Agitated
Agony
Alert
Alienated
Alive
Almighty
Alone
Amazed
Ambiguous
Ambitious
Ambivalent
Amused
Angry
Annoyed
Anxious
Appreciated
Apprehensive
Ashamed
Astonished
Astounded
Awed

Bad
Bashful
Beautiful
Belittled
Betrayed
Bewildered
Bitchy
Bitter
Blamed
Blissful
Blocked
Bold
Bored
Bothered
Brave
Burdened

Calm
Capable
Captivated
Cautious
Challenged
Charmed
Cheated
Cheerful
Cherished
Childish

Clever
Combative
Comfortable
Committed
Competitive
Concerned
Condemned
Confident
Conflicted
Confused
Conspicuous
Consumed
Contented
Contrite
Controlled
Cramped
Creative
Cruel
Crummy
Crushed
Culpable
Curious

Deceitful
Defeated
Defiant
Dejected
Delighted
Delirious
Depressed
Desirous
Despair
Destructive
Determined
Devastated
Different
Diffident
Diminished
Dirty
Disappointed
Discontented
Discouraged
Disgusted
Disorganized
Disoriented
Dissatisfied
Distracted
Distraught
Distressed
Distrustful
Disturbed
Divided
Dominated
Domineering
Doubtful
Down
Downtrodden
Drained
Driven
Dubious
Dumb

Ecstatic
Edgy
Elated
Electrified
Embarrassed
Empty
Enchanted
Encouraged
Endangered
Energetic
Enervated
Engrossed
Engulfed
Enjoy
Enlightened
Enraged
Enthusiastic
Envious
Euphoric
Evil
Excited

Fascinated
Fawning
Fearful
Flat
Flirtatious
Flustered
Foolish
Forgetful
Fragmented
Frantic
Free
Fretful
Friendly
Frightened
Frustrated
Full
Funny
Furious
Fury

Gay
Glad
Grateful
Gratified
Great
Greedy
Groovy
Grouchy
Guilty
Gullible

Happy
Hated
Hateful
Heavenly
Helpful
Helpless
High
Homesick
Honored
Hopeful
Hopeless
Horrible
Horrified
Hostile
Humble
Hurt

Ignorant
Ignored
Immortal
Impatient
Important
Imposed on
Impressed
Impulsive
Inadequate
Incomplete
Indifferent
Infantile
Infatuated
Infuriated
Insane
Insensitive
Inspired
Interested
Intimidated
Involved
Irritated
Isolated

Jealous
Jittery
Jolly
Joyful
Joyous
Jubilant
Jumpy

Keen
Kicky
Kind
Kinky

Laconic
Lazy
Lecherous
Left out
Let down
Lethargic
Licentious
Lighthearted
Limited
Listless
Lonely
Longing
Lost
Lousy
Loved
Loving
Low
Ludicrous
Lustful

Mad
Marvelous
Maudlin
Mean
Meek
Melancholy
Mellow
Miserable
Mistreated
Mistrusted
Misunderstood
Mixed up
Modest
Morose
Mystical
Mystified

Naughty
Needy

Negative
Neglected
Nervous
Nice
Nifty
Numb
Nutty

Obsessed
Odd
Opposed
Oppressed
Optimistic
Outraged
Overburdened
Overwhelmed

Pain
Pained
Panicked
Parsimonious
Pathetic
Patient
Peaceful
Perplexed
Persecuted
Perturbed
Pessimistic
Petrified
Phony
Picked on
Pissed-off
Pity
Pleasant
Pleased
Positive
Precarious
Preoccupied
Pressured
Pretty
Prim
Prissy
Productive
Proud
Pushed
Puzzled

Quarrelsome
Queer
Quiet

Rage
Rapture
Rebellious
Refreshed
Regretful
Rejected
Rejuvenated
Relaxed
Relieved
Remorse
Remorseful
Renewed
Resentful
Resigned
Responsible
Restless
Revenged
Reverent
Rewarded
Right
Righteous
Ripped-off
Rotten

Sad
Safe
Sated
Satisfied
Scared
Scattered
Screwed
Screwed up
Secure
Selfish
Selfless
Sensitive
Sensuous
Serene
Serious
Servile
Settled
Sexy
Shocked
Shitty
Sick
Silly
Skeptical
Slighted
Smothered
Sneaky
Sober
Solemn
Sophisticated

Sore
Sorrowful
Sorry
Spiteful
Squeezed
Strange
Strong
Stubborn
Stuck
Stuffed
Stumped
Stunned
Stupified
Stupid
Subordinated
Successful
Suffering
Superfluous
Superior
Sure
Surprised
Suspicious
Swamped
Sympathetic

Talkative
Tangled
Tempted
Tenacious
Tense
Tentative
Tenuous
Terrible
Terrific
Terrified
Testy
Threatened
Thwarted
Tired
Together
Torn
Tranquil
Trapped
Tremendous
Troubled
Turned off
Turned on

Ugly
Unafraid
Uncertain
Uncomfortable
Undermined
Unfortunate
Unhappy
Unimportant
Uninvolved
Unloved
Unlucky
Unnecessary
Unneeded
Unpleasant
Unproductive
Unsettled
Unsure
Unwanted
Upset
Uptight
Used
Useful
Useless

Vacant
Vague
Vain
Valued
Vapid
Vehement
Vicious
Victimized
Victorious
Vindictive
Violent
Vital
Vitality
Vivacious
Vulnerable

Wanted
Warm
Wasted
Weak
Weary
Wee
Weepy
Weird
Welcome
Well
Whimsical
Whole
Wicked
Wild
Willing
Wily

Wiry
Witless
Wonderful
Worldly
Worn out
Worried
Worthless
Worthwhile
Wound-up
Wretched

Yellow
Yucky

Zany
Zesty
Zippy
Zonked

Note. This is not an exhaustive list. Feel free to add to it.

BIBLIOGRAPHY

SPECIAL READINGS

Ivey, A., & Authier, J. (1978). *Microcounseling, innovations in interviewing, counseling, psychotherapy and psychoeducation*. Springfield, IL: Charles C. Thomas.

Rogers, C. (1979). The attitude and orientation of the counselor. In C. Rogers, *Client centered therapy*. Boston: Houghton Mifflin.

Rogers, C. R., & Skinner, B. F. (1956, November). Some issues concerning the control of human behavior—A symposium. *Science, 124*(3231), 1056–1066.

Seeman, J. (1986). Client centered therapy. In G. H. Shames & H. Rubin (Eds.), *Stuttering then and now* (pp. 316–334). Columbus, OH: Charles E. Merrill.

Travis, L. (1957). The unspeakable feelings of people with special reference to stuttering. In L. Travis (Ed.), *Handbook of speech pathology and audiology* (p. 938). Englewood Cliffs, NJ: Prentice-Hall.

REFERENCES

Boles, L. (1997). Conversation analysis as a dependent measure in communication therapy with four individuals with aphasia. *Asia Pacific Journal of Speech, Language, and Hearing, 2,* 233.

Boles, L., & Lewis, M. (1998). A qualitative analysis of solution focused couples therapy in an aphasic relationship. Submitted for publication to *Aphasiology,* pp. 43–61.

Carkhuff, R. (1969). *The counselor's contributions to facilitative processes.* (Mimeographed manuscript, Buffalo State University of New York, 1968. Cited in Carkhuff, R., *Helping and human relations.* New York: Holt, Reinhart & Winston.)

Carkhuff, R., & Berenson, B. (1976). *Teaching as treatment: An introduction to counseling and psychotherapy.* Amherst, MA: Human Resource Development.

de St.-Exupery, A. (1943). *The little prince* (pp. 65–71). New York: Harcourt, Brace, Jovanovich, Inc.

Dunlap, K. (1932). *Habits: Their making and unmaking.* New York: Liveright.

Flasher, L., & Fogle, P. (2004). *Counseling skills for speech-language pathologists and audiologists.* San Diego, CA: Singular Publishing Group.

Fromm-Reichmann, F. (1962). Patient–doctor relationship: Psychotherapist in the therapeutic process. In H. J. Bachrach (Ed.), *Experimental foundations of clinical psychology* (p. 582). New York: Basic Books.

Greenspoon, J. (1955). The reinforcing effect of two spoken sounds on the frequency of two responses. *American Journal of Psychology, 68,* 409–416.

Haan, N. (1977). *Coping and defending processes of self-environment organization.* New York: Academic Press.

Holland, A. (2002). The person with aphasia. In G. H. Shames & N. Anderson (Eds.), *Human communication disorders—An introduction* (6th ed., pp. 527–529). Boston, MA: Allyn & Bacon.

Hutchinson, B. B. (1979). Dialogues: Client–clinician communication. In B. B. Hutchinson, M. L. Hanson, & M. J. Mecham (Eds.), *Diagnostic handbook for speech pathology* (pp. 1–29). Baltimore, MD: Williams & Wilkins.

Ivey, A. (1983). *Intentional interviewing and counseling.* Monterey, CA: Brooks/Cole.

Ivey, A., & Authier, J., (1978). *Micro-counseling, innovations in interning, counseling: Psychotherapy, and psycho-education.* Springfield, IL: Charles C. Thomas.

Kagan, A., Winckel, J., & Shumway, E. (Producers). (1996). A film titled: *Supported conversation for aphasic adults, enhancing communication access*. Aphasia Center, North York, Ontario, Canada.

Kahn, R., & Cannell, C. (1957). *The dynamics of interviewing*. New York: John Wiley.

Kanfer, F., & Karoly, P. (1972). Self-control: A behavioristic excursion into the lion's den. *Behavior Therapy, 3,* 398–416.

Krasner, L. (1961). Studies of the conditioning of verbal behavior. In S. Saporta (Ed.), *Psycholinguistics: A book of readings* (pp. 75–96). New York: Holt, Rinehart & Winston.

Krasner, L. (1963). Reinforcement, verbal behavior, and psychotherapy. *American Journal of Orthopsychiatry, 33,* 601–613.

Lennard, H., & Bernstein, A. (1960). *The anatomy of psychotherapy*. New York: Columbia University Press.

Luterman, E. (1977). *Counseling parents of hearing impaired children*. Boston, MA: Little, Brown.

Luterman, E. (2001). *Counseling persons with communication disorders and their families*. Austin, TX: Pro-Ed.

Matarrazo, R. (1971). Research on the teaching and learning of psychotherapeutic skills. In A. Bergin & S. Garfield (Eds.), *Psychotherapy and behavior change* (pp. 895–924). New York: Wiley.

Matarrazo, J., Phillips, J., Wiens, A., & Saslow, G. (1965). Learning the art of interviewing: A study of what beginning students do and their patterns of change. *Psychotherapy: Theory, Research, and Practice, 2,* 49–60.

Payne, K., & Taylor, O. (2000). Multicultural influences on human communication. In G. H. Shames & N. Anderson, (Eds.), *Human communication disorders—An introduction* (6th ed., pp. 106–140). Boston, MA: Allyn & Bacon.

Pennebaker, J. (1990). *Opening up—The healing power of confiding in others*. New York: William Morrow.

Reik, T. (1949). *Listening with the third ear* (p. vii). New York: Farrar, Strauss.

Rogers, C. (1942). *Counseling and psychotherapy*. Boston, MA: Houghton-Mifflin.

Rogers, C. (1972). *Patterns of processes that take place in encounter groups. Information Cassette Series*. Chicago: Instructional Dynamics, Inc.

Rollin, W. J. (1987). *The psychology of communication disorders in individuals and their families*. Englewood Cliffs, NJ: Prentice-Hall.

Rollin, W. J. (2000). *Counseling individuals with communication disorders: Psychodynamic and family aspects*. Oxford, England: Butterworth-Heinemann.

Rotter, J. B. (1966). Generalized expectancies for internal vs. external control reinforcement. *Psychological Monographs* (Whole No. 609, pp. 1–28).

Salzinger, K. (1959). Experimental manipulation of verbal behavior: A review. *Journal of General Psychology, 61,* 65–94.

Salzinger, K., & Pisoni, S. (1957). *Reinforcement of affect responses of schizophrenics during the clinical interview*. Paper read at the annual meeting of the Eastern Psychological Association.

Schweitzer, A. (1965). *Reverence for life* (pp. 6–7). New York: Philosophical Library.

Shames, G. H. (1969). Verbal reinforcement during therapy interviews with stutterers. In B. Gray & E. England (Eds.), *Stuttering and the conditioning therapies* (pp. 99–114). Monterey, CA: Monterey Institute for Speech and Hearing.

Shames, G. H. (1993). *Clinical application manual. The sustained phonation feedback method of therapy for stuttering* (pp. 53–54).

Shames, G. H. (2000). *Counseling the communicatively disabled and their families—A manual for clinicians*. Boston, MA: Allyn & Bacon.

Shames, G., & Egolf, D. (1976). Verbal conditioning of desirable content and punishment of undesirable content during clinical interviews with stutterers. In G. H. Shames & D. Egolf

(Eds.), *Operant conditioning and the management of stuttering* (pp. 112–116). Englewood Cliffs, NJ: Prentice-Hall.

Shames, G. H., & Florance, C. F. (1980). *Stutter free speech: A goal for therapy*. Columbus, OH: Charles E. Merrill.

Shames, G., & Honeygosky, R. (1976). The conditioning of verbal expressions of anger. In G. H. Shames & D. Egolf (Eds.), *Operant conditioning and the management of stuttering* (pp. 112–116). Englewood Cliffs, NJ: Prentice-Hall.

Shames, G., & Johnson, C. (1976). Verbal conditioning of decisiveness and decision-making content in the responses of stutterers during clinical interviews. In G. H. Shames & D. Egolf (Eds.), *Operant conditioning and the management of stuttering* (pp. 112–116). Englewood Cliffs, NJ: Prentice-Hall.

Shipley, K. G. (1992). *Interviewing and counseling in communicative disorders, principles and procedures* (pp. 64–67). New York: Macmillan.

Skinner, B. F. (1953). *Science and human behavior*. New York: Macmillan.

Skinner, B. F. (1957). *Verbal behavior*. New York: Appleton-Century-Crofts.

Strupp, H. (1962). Patient–doctor relationship: Psychotherapist in the therapeutic process. In H. J. Bachrach (Ed.), *Experimental foundations of clinical psychology*. New York: Basic Books.

Strupp, H. (1972). On the technology of psychotherapy. *Archives of General Psychiatry, 26*, 270–278.

Sullivan, H. S. (1970). *The psychiatric interview*. New York: W. W. Norton.

Truax, C. (1966). Effective ingredients in psychotherapy: An approach to unraveling the patient–therapist interaction. In G. Stollak, B. Guerney, Jr., & M. Rothberg (Eds.), *Psychotherapy research: Selected readings* (pp. 586–594). Chicago: Rand.

Truax, C. (1967). A scale for the rating of accurate empathy. In C. Rogers, E. Gendlin, D. Kiesler, & C. Truax (Eds.), *The therapeutic relationship and its impact. A study of psychotherapy with schizophrenics* (pp. 555–568). Madison: University of Wisconsin Press.

Truax, C. (1972). The meaning and reliability of accurate empathy ratings: A rejoinder. *Psychological Bulletin, 77*, 397–399.

Wiig, E., & Secord, W. (1998). Language disabilities in school-age children and youth. In G. Shames, E. Wiig, & W. Secord (Eds.), *Human communication disorders—An introduction* (pp. 225–226). Boston, MA: Allyn & Bacon.

Wolf, S., & Wolf, C. (1975). *The counseling skills evaluation* (film).

Wolpe, J. (1986). Systematic desensitization based on relaxation. In G. H. Shames & H. Rubin (Eds.), *Stuttering then and now* (pp. 335–359). Columbus, OH: Charles E. Merrill.

AUTHOR INDEX

SUBJECT INDEX

G

H

I

L

M

N

O

P

R

S

T

V, W